I Have to Get Some Things off My Chest

Venecia Butler

CROSSBOOKS

CrossBooks™
A Division of LifeWay
1663 Liberty Drive
Bloomington, IN 47403
www.crossbooks.com
Phone: 1-866-879-0502

First published by CrossBooks 6/20/2013

ISBN: 978-1-4627-2911-1 (sc)
ISBN: 978-1-4627-2912-8 (e)

Library of Congress Control Number: 2013910976

Printed in the United States of America.

This book is printed on acid-free paper.

Edited by: Eddie Burkhalter and Kay Kisor
Illustrations by: Scott Clarke

Table of Contents

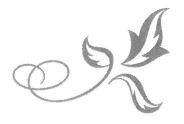

1 Peter 1: 6-7
New International Version (NIV)

6. In this you greatly rejoice, though now for a little while you may have to suffer grief in all kinds of trials. 7. These have come so that your faith-of greater worth than gold, which perishes even though refined by fire-may be proved genuine and may result in praise, glory and honor when Jesus Christ is revealed.

Endorsements

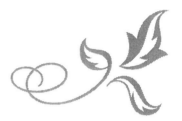

When Venecia told me about her book, my first thought was, "What a great title!" My second was what my pastor told me when I was a small child; "God deals the cards. Some of us get a good hand and some of us don't. What matters is how you play the hand he gives you."

I have known Venecia since 2006 and have witnessed her journey through surgery, radiation, chemo and endocrine therapy. Venecia has played with humor, courage and a strong desire to survive.

Our hope is that patients, their families and friends will find this book to be an inspiration.

Ellen Spremulli, MD

It's a hard thing to try and describe Venecia Butler. You'd just have to know her, I suppose, to know how funny she is and how strong. Meet her once and you know how much she cares about other people and that's why I think she wrote this book. It's because she has a passion for people who have cancer and those close to them. It's because she wanted to make their lives easier, to help them through the tough days just like when she'd put on a Tyler Perry movies in the chemo room. If you've got cancer, or know someone who has, this book can help. And if you ask Venecia, it wouldn't hurt to turn off The Price Is Right and throw Tyler Perry in the DVD player.

Eddie Burkhalter

Early on in 2012, I was favored by God to meet an amazing woman. A woman I have come to love and cherish. Resolute yet cautious, convivial yet staid, enervated yet strengthened; she has battled and won the beast named Cancer three times. She finished her third crusade last year and has taken the blessing of victory in Jesus onto the road speaking…making people laugh and feel courageous in their own battles.

Her attitude has been one of ferocious faith in our Father. In her, I have seen an example of "fighting the good fight." (1 Tim 6:12) Recently she learned the monster had returned for a fourth time. When others would raise their white flag to forfeit or accept defeat, she has chosen to forge ahead, clothed in the Armor of God, (Eph 6:10-18) for His glory, she prepares for yet another war within her body. Gaffed to face what is necessary in her refinement, she praises her Father. (2 Tim 3:17, 1 Pet 1:6-7)

There have been several women who have been examples to me, but I never personally met a woman who made me desire to totally transform my thought process…the friend she has been called to bear within her person has been an illumination of Christ. I have witnessed His strength in her. Jehovah Rapha (The Lord our Healer) dwells within my friend, Venecia Butler. Praise God that she is a reflection of Him in her season of trials. (Ecc 3:1-14) May she be abundantly rewarded for yet another time to tear to down. May 2013 be "A Time to Heal." The world needs more women like her in it!!!!!!

Tammy Moss

In my 23 years of oncology nursing, I have not come across a patient with such rib-tickling humor as Venecia. Finding such humor in cancer treatment is a hard thing to do. Venecia has shared her personal story on the pages of this book and made her story come to life. If you or a family member is experiencing cancer, I recommend this book to lighten the mood.

Wendy Watson, RN, OCN

Venecia Butler has lived with breast cancer for almost seven years. It has been a great privilege for me to serve as one of her physicians during that time. Venecia suffered through all the shock and disappointment that all patients feel when diagnosed with breast cancer; surgery, chemotherapy, radiation therapy and then recurrence of breast cancer can overwhelm a strong person. Venecia is one who overcomes and has strong faith. I believe by God's grace, Venecia will live a long and fruitful life.

Roderick G Johnson, MD

I have to Get Some Thing's off My Chest, is a witty account about the journey of being diagnosed, treated, and living with breast cancer. The dry humor that Venecia uses, referring to radiation treatments as visiting the nuclear spa, is a way for her to cope but also to put a smile on the face of someone having their own "spa" treatment. It is honest, brave and demonstrates her strength in a situation that has caused so many others to surrender.

Candi Fisher

We are excited what God is going to do by putting your life experiences to paper. When you have walked the walk, it comes across as such a blessing to the reader. Thank God for you and sharing a slice (pardon the pun) of your life.

We love you,

Mom and Dad

Dedication

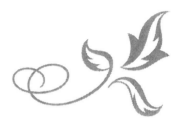

To my great parents, Charles and Sandra Benefield; thank you for all the support you have given me all my life. I am sorry I have brought you back from Tennessee so much in the last seven years.

To my sister Randa; you have been the best caretaker and cheerleader a person could have. You have gone the second and third mile for me over and over again.

To my brother in law Bobby Joe; thanks for shaving my head and always being there.

To my friends and the City of Piedmont; I am humbled by your love and support.

To Nathan and Chelsea; I am so proud to be your mother. You are my heart and I will continue to fight for you.

To Curtis; you have been so faithful to stand beside me and be the rock that holds our family together.

I love you all very much!

In memory of; my Great Aunt Mary Ruth and my grandmothers Edna Bragg and Lillian Benefield; you left me a legacy of courage, strength and honor. I miss you very much.

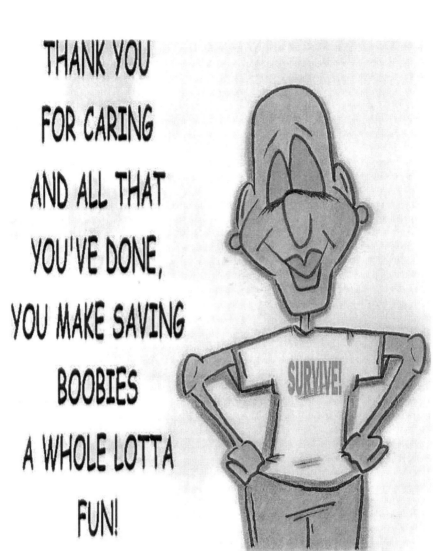

Acknowledgements

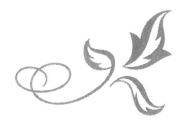

To my Lord and Saviour Jesus Christ – I am grateful for your love and honored that You chose me to battle cancer and to be a speaker and a writer. I hope I have made you proud.

Eddie Burkhalter – Thank you for helping me format and edit this book and taking time to tell my story in the newspaper.

Kay Kisor – You were a great English teacher, sorry I didn't pay attention in your class. Thank you for editing this book and making it as good as it can be.

Scott Clarke at Crabby Cards – Thank you for allowing me to use your great illustrations.

Steel Magnolias – Thank you for all the snacks and drinks, and all you provide for the chemo patients.

Kim Compton – I am amazed how God orchestrated our friendship. Thank you for not letting me wallow in self pity and making me get out of bed.

Kelly Stewart – Thank you for making me laugh and helping me share my story. Without you there would be no "Crap".

Dana Cupo– Thanks for all your help and for all the encouragement you have given me.

Belinda Clanton – Thanks for going the extra mile and having me a Crap shirt made. Because of you "Crap" is worldwide.

Becky Stewart – Thanks for being my "handler" and taking time everyday at 8:30 a.m. to call and pray with me, and all your support.

Kayron Berry – Thanks for bringing us all together for Lesa's memorial and the great memories. Because of you we are the Yayas!

The Yayas – Thank you for your friendship, and all the laughs and prayers.

Jacksonville Christian Academy and Jacksonville Christian Child Development Center – Thank you my co-workers, and all the teachers and students for supporting and praying for me, and loving Nathan and Chelsea. Marla Morales – You were at great boss!

To all my Doctors and nurses – Thank you for all of the great care you have given me.

Last but not least, my family – Curtis, Nathan, Chelsea, Mom and Dad, Randa and Bobby Joe, Shirley and Wayne, Robert and Etoice– God has blessed me with the best family. Thank you for loving me through it. I love you!

Foreword

It is hard to understand why kind, funny, good, honest, God loving people often seem to find themselves traveling the difficult paths of life. Maybe it is because God knows they have the faith and grace to make it through the hardship and heartache and succeed in whatever it is they are meant to do and to be. Somehow they are able to reach deep inside their souls and find the strength to use their pain for a greater cause.

From the beginning, I knew Venecia Butler was different than most of my other patients. Venecia is one of the patients that I will remember for all my life. For one thing, she is funny, hilariously funny. For another, she is brutally honest. It has never been hard to figure out what is on her mind. If she is scared, she will tell you. If she is mad, she will tell you that too. Venecia has that positive energy and doesn't bottle it. She has a strength that could only come from God. She connects like a sister, like a best friend. In watching her, I can see myself, my siblings and my best friends.

After I moved away from North Alabama, she contacted me to let me know that her cancer had recurred. I was very sad but not surprised. It seems that all too often, it is the special people like her that are asked to travel the most difficult paths. Venecia Butler is a special person.

At her clinic visits, we used to talk about her book. I wanted her to write a book about her life after being diagnosed with cancer. As a doctor and a friend, I am so grateful that she is telling her story. She is a light in the dark that will help others find their way.

Dr. Stephanie Fussell

1 Corinthians 1:27

But God hath chosen the foolish things of the world to confound the wise; and God hath chosen the weak things of the world to confound the things which are mighty.

To God be the glory!

Introduction

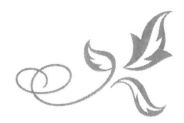

If you've picked up this book, you or someone close to you may have heard the awful words, "its cancer". I'd love to say that everything's going to be all right, but honestly, it's going to be a battle unwinnable alone.

To begin, the strength and peace that comes from a personal relationship with God will help you get through the difficult road ahead. And it's important to surround yourself with as many unselfish people as you can find.

I did not set out to be a writer. This book is my first, and I believe I was ordained by God to write it. I am thankful I was told in 2006 that I had cancer because this news changed my life: I appreciate everyone and everything in my life now, and I realize just how fragile and short life can be.

I chose to laugh at cancer, not that it's funny to see people - myself included - sitting in a chemo room fighting to live, but laughter gives you power. Laughter lifts the spirit, and cancer victims need both power and spirit to win this battle.

I hope my experience with cancer will help you understand what those like me go through, all the emotions we feel and what it means to live with this disease. I hope that you'll laugh - maybe for the first time - at cancer.

So if you would, turn the page and walk with me on my journey...

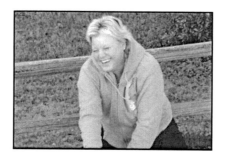

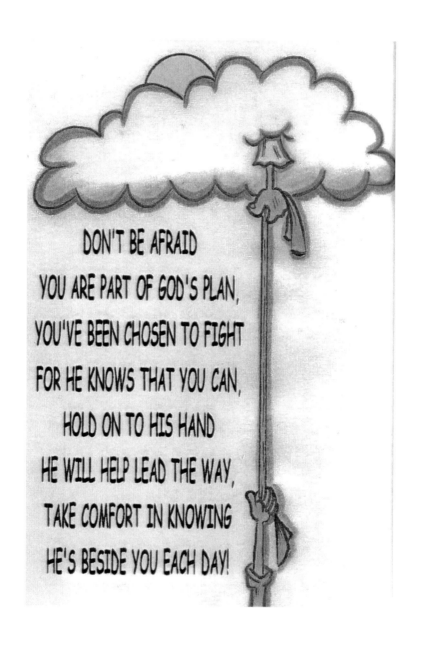

February 2006...The Day My Life Changed

All people who have had cancer can tell you what was happening in their lives when they were diagnosed. When you receive that news, some things in your life become much clearer. When I got the news, I had been married to Curtis for sixteen years and was a mother to two wonderful children: Nathan, eleven and Chelsea, ten. Ever since Nathan was in second grade I had home-schooled both of my children. It was the best time of my life. Looking back, I am so thankful God gave me that special time with my children.

To begin, let me back up to my hysterectomy in January 2005. After the procedure I was prescribed hormones, like the majority of women, for the next year, I took Premarin, which I renamed the "Miracle-Gro of cancer cells," because I was told that the cancer cells in my body had multiplied as a result of my usage. I was forty-two years old and I had cancer.

It was not unusual for me to have breast pain, and I was well aware of the risk of taking hormones, but in February, 2006, I felt a lump in my breast. I wasn't alarmed because I was told a tender lump was usually not cancer. I believed these lumps were typically cysts...Lie! I wish you could hear me scream, "It is a *lie!*"

Here is what I want you to learn from me: The minute you feel a lump, get yourself to the doctor for a mammogram...ASAP. Okay, back to my story.

Every day I would feel to see if the knot was still there. Yep. It was still there. I knew I had a mammogram scheduled for April, so I waited...*Big mistake!*

Remember: Do not wait if you feel a lump. Go immediately to your doctor.

When April finally arrived, I went for my annual mammogram. After seven days I received a phone call that the mammogram was abnormal and to come in for a magnification mammogram.

For people unfamiliar with this process, let me share. They get a tractor-trailer truck and run over your boob, flattening it to the width of a piece of paper. You are unable to breathe as a truck is on top of your boob, but they still feel the need to tell you not to breathe. Well of course I won't, because I can't. The boob slowly goes back to normal, and you wait for results. The tests were sent to Birmingham, and after a few days I received a call to see a surgeon for a biopsy. My results were not good.

Side Note for God!

I love looking back and seeing how God was taking care of me the whole time. Before all the discussions about cancer had begun, God was moving me to put Nathan and Chelsea back in school. We had an interview at Jacksonville Christian Academy. I had perfect peace that this was where they belonged, but of course God already knew that! He knew what I was facing and took care of everything.

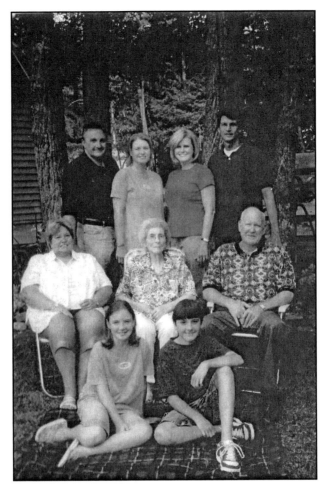

My family in 2006

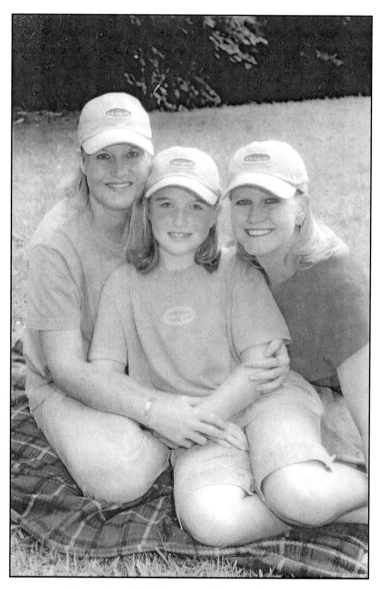

Randa, Chelsea and me in 2006

Biopsy

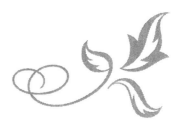

On Thursday, May 18, 2006, I met Dr. Johnson who did my biopsy. Thankfully my Mom, Sandra Benefield, and Chelsea were able to stay in the room with me. I had a stereotactic biopsy.

Let me describe this procedure for you. There is a table with a hole cut out. You put on your paper gown, lay down flat, and insert boob A into the hole. Then a machine underneath comes up to flatten boob A once again. This time they did give a shot to deaden boob A. Then the doctor gets on a contraption they use to roll under a car to change the oil.

Dr. Johnson rolled under my boob to begin the biopsy process. My poor mother and Chelsea were watching the whole process with their mouths hanging open and eyes wide open. Dr. Johnson removed a piece of the tumor. After the biopsy, Dr. Johnson talked to me about the different options I would have if it was cancer. The mass was big, going across my breast and under my arm, and he thought I would be able to have a lumpectomy followed by seven weeks of radiation. He sent the biopsy to the hospital, and I waited for the results.

Side Note for God

The next day, May 19, was my forty-second birthday and Chelsea's dress rehearsal for her dance recital. I saw Kim Compton at the rehearsal, a high school friend I hadn't seen in several years. We had been really close friends, but as friends do, over the years we had drifted apart. However, God had my back again and was putting her back into my life.

Kim had two children: Calley and Caden, whom she had decided to put into JCA also, and Chelsea and Calley would be in the same grade! God was on it for me and my children. Chelsea and Calley met that night and remain best friends to this day.

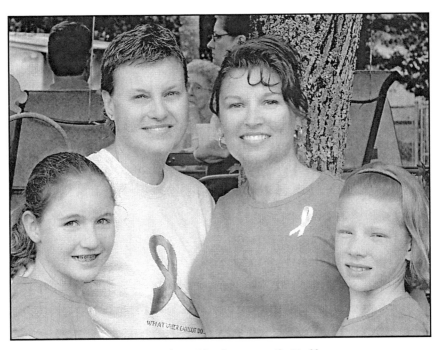

Kim and I Chelsea and Calley

The Talk

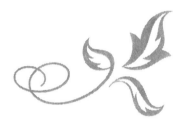

When Dr. Johnson's nurse called with my biopsy results, I could tell by her voice that something was wrong. She told me that Dr. Johnson wanted me to come in the next day so he could talk with me. Since Curtis would be at work at the time of the appointment, he planned to meet me there. My daddy, Charles Benefield, rode to the doctor's office with me. Once we got there, they took us into a room with really comfortable chairs. I guess they want you to be comfortable when they are going to tell you something bad.

I was really expecting to hear "lumpectomy, and seven weeks of radiation." Instead, I heard "infiltrating ductular carcinoma" which meant a radical mastectomy, eight chemo treatments, seven weeks of radiation, and, according to Dr. Johnson, "the worst year of my life."

At that moment I felt as if I was floating above myself, looking down at the doctor, Curtis, and Dad. It was such a surreal moment. People were talking, but it didn't seem real.

They all turned into Charlie Brown's teacher, and all I heard was, "Wah wah woh wah wah." The cancer was invasive and aggressive, but Dr. Johnson was so sweet,. talking to me like a grandfather telling his granddaughter she was very sick.

I had heard other people say it, but I can verify it: life as you know it stops, and everything changes. Your life is taken over by doctors. The song "Live Like You Were Dying" became so real to me that day. It's amazing how your will to live kicks in when you have something inside you that wants to kill you.

Dr. Johnson said I couldn't wait long to have the surgery. I was totally overwhelmed. I just wanted to be by myself and try to understand what was happening to me. Daddy was with me, but I told him I didn't want to talk. Being the great and understanding daddy he is, he didn't say anything except, "Honey, do you want me to drive?" Unfortunately for my dad, I did not let him drive. My driving on the way home scared him to death. His knuckles turned white as he hung on for dear life while I drove recklessly home. All I wanted to do was to get home and be by myself before talking to Nathan and Chelsea. I dropped Daddy off at Randa's so I could be by myself before seeing Nathan and Chelsea. How I really was dreaded telling them! They were at Mother's house watching the *American Idol* finale. Since I had been truthful with them the entire time, they knew my appointment with the doctor was to find out if I had cancer. I arrived my mom's at eight o'clock, and Nathan rode home with me while Chelsea rode with her dad.

I'll never forget when we got in the car, and he looked at me with those big brown eyes and said, "You have cancer, don't you, Momma?" Those words tore my heart out. I told him we would talk about it when we got home.

Talking with my children about this was the hardest thing I have ever done. I told them everything the doctor had said and what the next year would be like. As a mother, I didn't want my children to worry about me or see me in pain, so I told them I would not have chemothearpy if they didn't want me to. However, I was a fighter, and I was willing to do whatever to live for them.

Chelsea asked, "Are you going to lose your hair?" I replied, "yes". Nathan sat there with tears in his eyes and asked me if I was going to die. My throat had a knot growing larger and larger. How was I supposed to answer that? I told them to pray for me. They didn't hesitate to come over to me, laid their hands on my head, and prayed. Both children said the sweetest prayer for me, giving me a sense of peace. Yep, I have two awesome children.

I called my pastor to pray for me the next day. I had people praying for me to be healed. I was quite sure no surgery or chemo was needed, and I knew God would go along with my plan. It sounded like a good plan to me. Because I was so sure God was on board with my plan, I called Deborah, Dr. Johnson's nurse, and told her the only way I would schedule surgery was if they would give me another mammogram before I had to have a mastectomy.

I was thinking I wanted them to be blessed by my healing and see that I no longer needed the surgery. She agreed and since surgery was scheduled for Friday, the mammogram was to be done on Wednesday

I found strength in the strangest place, sitting outside in a green chair. That's where I had long talks with Kim and where I felt closest to God. The one thing I did not want to do was chemo. I wasn't upset about having a mastectomy, but going through chemo was something I adamantly opposed. When I found out about my cancer, I came up with an alternative plan: I thought I'd just get a cross tattooed on my breast and ask God to take care of everything. No one liked that idea but me, so I decided to go along with the mastectomy. Dr. Johnson said I would have seven weeks of radiation for sure, and if it had moved into my lymph nodes, I would have to do chemo.

Wednesday arrived, and it was time for the mammogram that would show everyone God had healed my tumor. They showed me the picture. I saw the tumor; hence, even before Deborah called, I knew it was still there.

But I was good with my boob being cut off. In fact, I wanted both of them cut off. I wanted the cancer out and to move on with my life. Dr. Johnson said it would be - in his words - "overkill" for both boobs to be removed, but I still wasn't planning to go through chemo. After seeing family and friends go through it, I did not want to experience it at all.

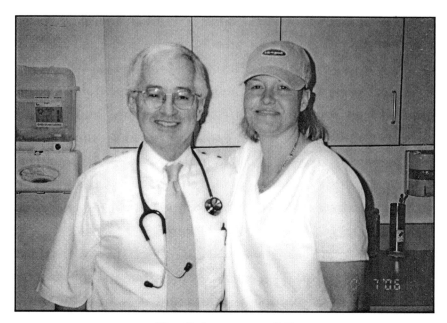

Dr. Johnson and I

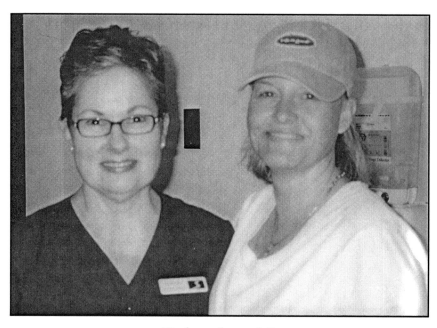

Deborah and I

CANCER WILL
CHALLENGE BOTH
BODY AND SOUL,
THE DESTRUCTION
AND SCARS MAKE
YOU FEEL LESS
THAN WHOLE,
BUT GOD DOESN'T
LEAVE US TO
BATTLE ALONE,
OUR PRAYERS ARE
THE THREAD OF
WHICH MIRACLES
ARE SEWN,
YOUR PRAYERS WILL
BE TAKEN TO GOD
AND BE GIVEN,
AND THE ANGELS
THAT TAKE THEM
ARE WEARING
PINK RIBBONS!

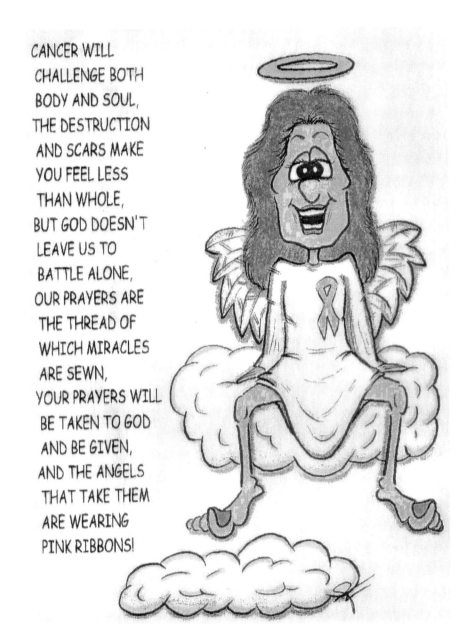

My First Mastectomy

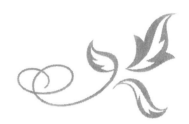

Iwent for my lab work and was set for surgery the next day, June 2, 2006. I arrived at the hospital at six o'clock that morning and waited forever before someone saw me. Luckily, my family was waiting with me in the room.

I looked at Randa and told her to go get me a sharpie. It was time to design a headstone for my breast. My last farewell to boob A. I wrote "RIP 1964-2006" on my breast. It made me smile to think of Dr. Johnson laughing when he started the surgery. Papa Johnson was a little serious, and I felt it was my duty to loosen him up.

Finally, a guy named Jerry came to get me and take me back to have my sentinal node. His wild do-rag caught my eye. I said, "Hey, Jerry. I like your do-rag, and I am going to need it in a couple of months."

I asked him to give it to me of course, and Jerry just laughed and said he couldn't part with it because it was his favorite do-rag. I Looked Jerry dead in the eye and told him if he didn't give it me that God would make it unravel, and every time he looked in the mirror he'd see my face. Not that I believe in hexes or anything, but I was one-hundred percent sure God was in on all my plans. Surprisingly, Jerry held strong, rejected my plea, and wheeled me down for my sentinal node.

I was totally unaware of the pain awaiting me. A long needle was used to inject dye all around my nipple. Deborah,the nurse, held my hand as my feet pressed against the wall. I looked at her with gritted teeth and said, "I think I am going to push a hole in the wall." It's still too painful to describe.

Finally it was over. When Jerry came back to get me, I asked again for the do-rag. Jerry said, "No, Mrs. Butler. You're not going to get my do rag."

Jerry took me back to my room to wait for surgery, and my pastor, Kent Mattox, came by to see me. Before he left, he asked if he could do anything for me, and I shared the story of Jerry and the do-rag.

Hours later, I smiled as they wheeled me back into my room after surgery; On my bed lay Jerry's do-rag. Kent showed me what it means to go the extra mile for someone. Having walked the halls searching for Jerry, Kent discovered he had left for the day. Undeterred, he then called a member of our church, Danny, who worked in the physical therapy department. Kent pled with Danny to locate Jerry and obtain the much desired do-rag. Danny went to Jerry's house to ask about the do-rag and Jerry asked nervously, "Did Mrs. Butler send you over here?"

I would have loved to see the expression on Jerry's face, and I often wonder if he thought for a moment his curse was coming true. Danny told Jerry that Kent wanted to get the do-rag for me and asked what it would take. Jerry said it would cost $50.

Kent paid him, and Danny chased him down! The extra mile, indeed!

Not long afterward, Dr. Johnson came in and told me the cancer had moved to my lymph nodes. All I could think was, "Why did I not go to the doctor sooner?" I was furious at myself for waiting until April for that mammogram.

Remember ladies: the second you feel a lump, go straight to the doctor and have a mammogram.

Oh well. I couldn't go back.

I did really well after surgery. I took a lot of pain medicine and phenergan, so I was in and out of it for most of the first day. When I was out of it, we were laughing and having a good time. Infact, It got so out of hand the nurses had to come tell us we were making too much noise. They said we needed to quiet down because there were sick people there.

My sister Randa and her husband Bobby Joe went to Spencer's Gifts and bought me a pair of boobs. If somone buys you boobs after yours are cut off, you put them on, especially if you're on major pain medicine.

A sweet lady from the American Cancer Society came by to talk to me, and with a confused look on her face, she asked, "Is this Mrs. Butler's room who had a mastectomy?"

We all burst into laughter. I'm the only person who comes out of a mastectomy surgery with bigger boobs than when I went in. *Awkward moment for her.*

I was sent home with two drain tubes, and I quickly discovered walking around with tubes hanging from your chest is a pain. I manuevered around the house with the lovely tubes for four days. Dr. Johnson told me I had to heal before chemo could start.

Time To Counsel With God

I did awesome physically, but emotionally, it was another story. During my disturbed period, I did some brave, stupid, courageous, and crazy things.

As a thunderstorm approached one night, I decided I'd *counsel* with God. The mother instinct in me gathered up my two precious children, and I said, "Ya'll go play in your room while mom sits outside in the thunderstorm." It is okay for mom to sit in a thunderstorm, but children should never do this.

They thought I had lost my mind. I had already *told* God I did not want to go through chemo, but I wanted to make sure He understood *I did not* want to go through chemo. I knew He could have taken the cancer away before it advanced this far, and that He had a plan, but I've always been hard-headed.

Sitting in my green metal chair out in the thunderstorm I said to God, "I will give you ten minutes to strike me with lightning."

I wasn't scared, just soaking wet. Lightning struck all around, but it never struck me. Ten minutes passed and not a single lightning bolt came my way. *Okay, I get it God. I am going through chemo.*

I realized for the first time I wasn't scared of death; I was ready to fight cancer and win. The fight with big C had begun.

I met with Dr. Fussell June 21 and felt comfortable with her and the staff. I had a MUGA scan, bone scan, CAT scan and a PET scan. Since I could only use my right arm for blood work, every inch of it was poked to get blood. My arm looked like it had been run over by a car. My port was put in nine days later, on June 30. After unsuccessfully attempting to insert the IV into my right arm, the anesthia Dr. finally put it in my foot.

However, the anesthia doctor also had a cool do-rag, white with red hearts; he was more cooperative than Jerry, giving me his do-rag after I asked just once. They rolled me into surgery wearing my new do rag on my head.

Each day was filled with dread because of the impending chemo treatments. It's hard to get excited about the prospect of filling your body with poison. My first treatment was July 11.

Once I shared with my research nurse Wendy the incident about sitting in my metal chair underneath a lightning storm. Since she didn't know me or my mental state very well, she told Dr. Fussell all about it, and while I was being hooked up to chemo, Dr. Fussell sent me the phone number for a psychiatrist! I laughed to myself wondering what the psychiatrist would think of me tatotting a cross on my boob and not doing chemo. Wendy soon learned a psychiatrist couldn't help me!

The next wonderful discovery was like a good news, bad news situation. The good news was I was young and healthy; the bad was that I'd require a stronger type of chemo. The first visit only lasted an hour-and-a-half. Emend, a nausea medicine costing $100 per pill, quickly became my best friend.

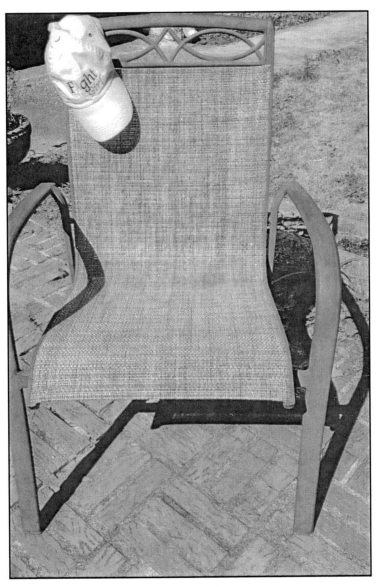

My Chair

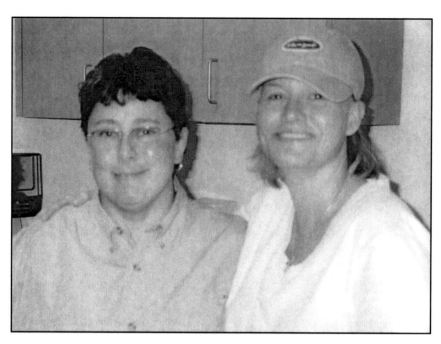

Dr. Fussell and I

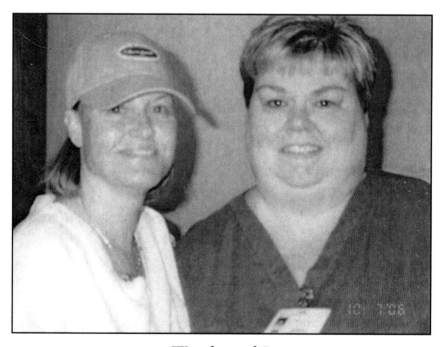

Wendy and I

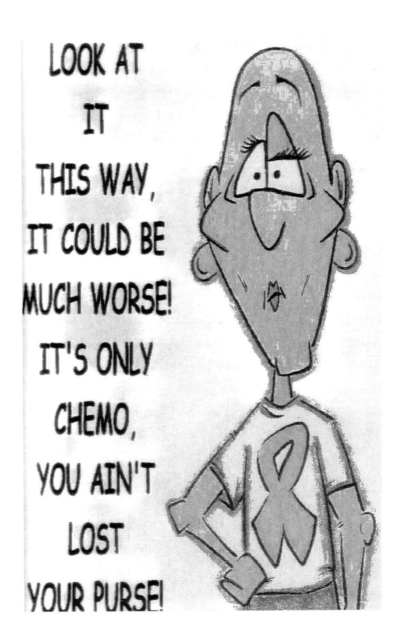

Red Devil

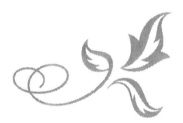

The chemo cocktail I was taking was called Adriamycin Cytoxan, also known as "red devil." It's a very aggressive, extremely toxic chemo treatment. It's red and is injected from a massive horse syringe.

The chemo nurse, dressed in cap, gown, and gloves, had to administer it by hand into my vein very slowly. Curious I asked, "Why are you going so slow?"

She replied that it could cause permanent heart damage or asphyxiation if put in too fast.

"Okey dokey! "Well slow it down then."

It was the weirdest sensation, the feeling of poison going through my body; it felt as if I were drifting away. After the treatment, the nurse told me to be sure to flush the toilet two to three times with the lid down, and wash my hands for 45 seconds. *And this is IN my body?*

I had four treatments with Red Devil. The day after chemo I was given a shot to rebuild my white blood cells. It kicked my butt and made me feel as if I'd come down with the flu.

The cancer chemo combination was enough to make me start a bucket list. I've always wanted a jeep, but Curtis would always say, "Not practical." I thought maybe since I had the big "C" he would get me one. *Wrongo!*

I needed to be in a jeep, to be riding around with the top down. Luckily, when one door closes, another one opens: Bobby Joe's brother let me borrow a jeep.

Driving in the jeep made me feel free. Loaded in the jeep, I'd search for as much mud as possible. Four-wheeling and dodging trees freed my mind of everything. It was the exact medicine I needed at that moment.

I had a strong desire to be out in nature. One day I floated the creek with Chelsea and Nathan. Some of my crazy stunts will have to remain in the "vault."

My nurse suggested that I get my hair cut short so that when it started falling out it wouldn't be so overwhelming. Sounded like a good idea, and my sister Randa was on it, immediately calling her stylist Kerry for an appointment. She gave me a very short-styled cut, but I didn't get to enjoy it for long.

On July 30, after only two treatments, I was washing my hair, and it began coming out by the handful. I was overcome with sadness. Out of all the things that had happened up to that point, losing my hair pushed me over the edge. It was the first time I'd cried.

Then my tears turned to anger and I was mad, the fight was on. Since I was diagnosed with cancer, I felt as though I had lost control. I would not allow cancer to determine when I would lose my hair. I was going to take my hair-not chemo. I picked up the phone and called Randa and Bobby Joe. They came over with dog clippers, and Bob shaved my head. I had already said "no wig!" so I learned how to tie on a do-rag, and life went on.

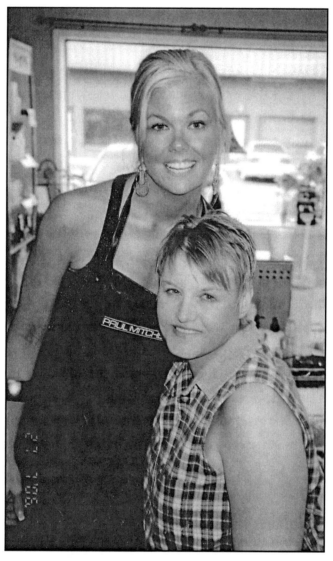

Kerry and my short hair cut

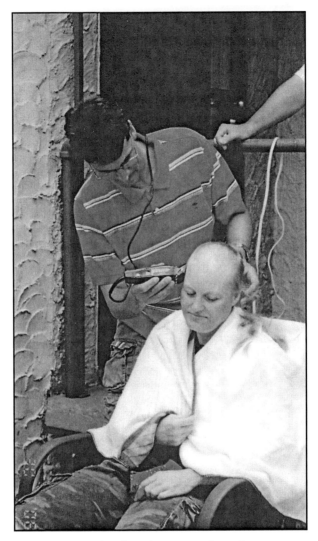

Bob shaving my head

My Weapons

The weapons I used were:

1. God
2. Laughter

3. Music

All three are very powerful.

God and Health

Jehovah Rophi

Exodus 15:26

I the Lord am your healer. (New English Bible)

...for I the Lord am thy physician. (Leeser)

...I am the Lord your life-giver. (Basic English)

...I am Yahweh thy physician. (Rotherham)

...I, Jehovah, am healing thee. (Young)

...For I, the Lord, make you immune to them (diseases). (Smith–Godspeed)

...I, the Lord, will bring thee only health.

Benefits of Laughter

1. Laughter helps the pituitary gland release its own pain surpressing opiates.
2. Lowers blood pressure.
3. Increases vascular blood flow and oxygenation of the blood.
4. Gives a workout to the diaphragm and abdomen, respiratory, facial, leg and back muscles.
5. Reduces certain stress hormones such as cortisol and adrenaline.
6. Increases the response of tumor and disease killing cells such as gamma-interferon and the cells.

7. Defends against respiratory infections...even the frequency of colds by immunoglobulin in saliva.
8. Increases memory and learning.
9. Improves alertness, creativity and memory.
10. *My favorite:* One laugh burns six calories and is egual to three spoonfuls of oat bran.

Benefits of Music

1. Manages pain.
2. Reduces stress.
3. Boosts immune system.
4. Encourages exercise.
5. Promotes sleep.
6. *My favorite:* Helps you drive faster and more reckless when going through chemo.

I would listen to praise music, everything from Hillsong. Then I'd go for a ride and listen to Kiss and Journey. "The Warrior" by Patti Smyth and "Survivor" by Destiny's Child became *my* songs. I'd drive like a bat out of hell because I knew I was going through chemo. No one wanted to ride with me.

I would tell them I knew where I'd be the next year, and ask, "Do you?" No one knew, so they didn't take a chance!

I've heard there are three types of sickness: Sickness to death, sickness to Chastisement and sickness to glorify God.

I was counting on the last.

My first goal at every chemo was to find the person that looked as though they had no hope and sit beside them. Nothing takes your mind off yourself like finding someone worse off. I would have them laughing before the nurse had my IV going.

My second goal was to get the television off "The Price is Right". The first goal was always easier to accomplish than the second. I was always the youngest one the room, so I'd put in a Tyler Perry play or movie, and my fellow chemo neighbors and I would laugh the whole time.

That brings me to my next point: The only positive thing I thought of when told I had cancer was that I'd lose weight... *Not*!

I was the only patient eating during chemo. I'd always hit the snack basket and refrigerator before being hooked up, and on my long days, I ordered pizza!

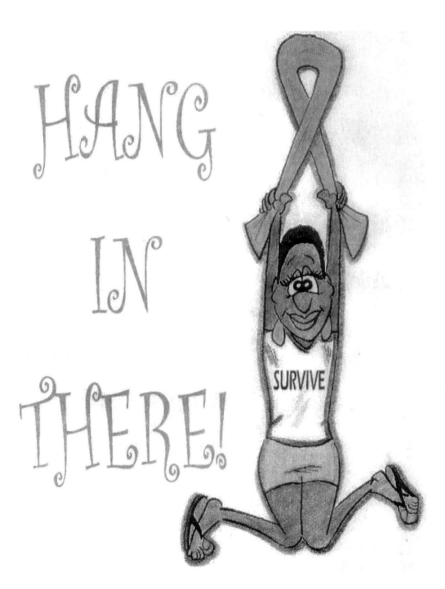

Chemo Brain

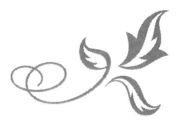

Technically called Cognitive Dysfunction, this condition is simply referred to as "chemo brain" to cancer patients. It's what can happen over time as the various toxins in chemotherapy, in their effort to kill cancer cells, make their way through the blood stream and the brain, disturbing normal functioning. Or in plain language, when the chemo causes the brain to forget how to think clearly, how to remember what you were just thinking, or what it was supposed to be doing. Or as I like to say, "Whobie dobie whatie?"

One day your mind is clear as a bell, and the next you feel as if your brain is in a fog. Remembering things becomes very difficult-not only little things, but big things as well. Things in general, like "what was I just saying?" or "what's the word for that thing you stick into food and then slide into your mouth?" or "I've been to this doctor a thousand times in the past two months, but for the life of me, I can't remember how to get there."

About that time, I was beginning to think that in addition to cancer, I now had Alzheimer's disease. But then, thanks to chemo Brain, I suddenly forgot what I was just thinking. I joke about it; I have to. If I didn't, it might scare me to death.

Advice for coping with chemo brain

1. Never lose your sense of humor.
2. Find ways to exercise your brain.

Anyway, where was I? Oh yeah...ways to deal with chemo brain.

3. Keep a Journal. I wrote my experiences, my fears, my frustrations – one: having to watch "The Price is Right"!
4. Never lose your Sense of Humor. (Oh, I forgot, that was number 1!)

During my treatment, my grandmother, Edna Bragg, was diagnosed with ovarian cancer. Two months later my dad was diagnosed with leukemia, and two weeks later he had open heart surgery. Needless to say, my mother was a basket case. Kim, being the supportive BFF, was determined I was not going to become depressed and wallow in self pity.

After one of my treatments, instead of going home and going to bed as I usually did, she wanted to get me out of the house. We went to UAB Hospital to see her co-worker Mack. Instead of parking in the parking deck, I had the great idea of just parking on the street, bad idea.

When we came out of hospital, we were on the opposite

side from where we came in. I had chemo brain, so I wasn't any good at remembering where we parked! After walking in the cold for almost an hour, we finally found the van. Needless to say, that was an adventure.

Randa always took me to get my shot the day after chemo. She also wanted to keep me up, so we'd go to Applebee's after the shot to eat and get a Blondie…nuff said. *Second reason I didn't lose weight.*

Third reason: Steroids. I hate them. I told Dr. Fussell I wasn't going to take them. She said, "Do you want to win?" *Gerrrrrr!* I was beginning to look like a sumo wrestler. All this chemo and I was still eating and not throwing up.

That's my God. Thankfully, He ignored my death request sitting in the lighting storm that day. Thank God for unanswered prayers!

I was doing so great with my chemo that I decided God was allowing me to go through this to help everybody else in chemo, and to help the nurses who took care of us. I took my mission to be positive and funny seriously. My answer to the question, "How are you feeling?" was always "Great!" Unfortunately, that wasn't everyone's response. I can't stand to be around negative people. I made it through the rest of my chemo treatments very well, with no hospital visits or sickness. I like to think my positive outlook was a major contributing factor.

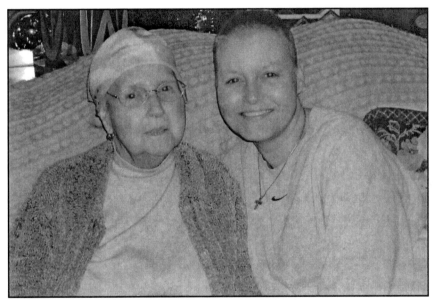

My Grandmother Bragg and I

The Nuclear Spa

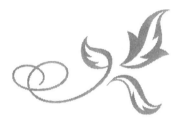

I started my "slow burn" at the Nuclear Spa, also known as radiation, in the middle of November. For those who have cancer and will be having radiation, there is no connection between therapeutic radiation and the types of radiation in bombs and nuclear reactors. Trust me; I did my research.

I had to take thirty-eight treatments. After going through chemo taking "red devil", I knew radiation would be a piece of cake. While I was waiting for my first treatment, I sat down next to a "Debbie Downer". She asked me what kind of cancer I had, and when I told her, she asked if it had moved to my lymph nodes. I said yes, and she responded, "Oh no! You know it will be back, probably in your lungs or brain."

Wow. Thanks for telling me. *Not!*

I was called back to see the doctor, and he marked my chest where I was to be zapped. I had to walk down a hallway to get to the radiation room so I became really good at tying my hospital gown by myself. After a week of tying, I said forget it, and would walk to the room with my gown untied. After months of taking my clothes off for doctors, I had no shame.

I drove myself to radiation every day. Daddy was at RMC in Gadsden, about thirty minutes away from RMC in Anniston, and so every day after radiation, I'd go and stay with him. He'd always be sitting in the recliner, so I would lie in the hospital bed. We both had no hair, and we freaked out a lot of nurses.

I did really great with the radiation, having no side effects or burns. It went great! I finished on December 23, 2006, and was very thankful to celebrate Christmas with my family. We'd been through a very rough year, but we were all still there.

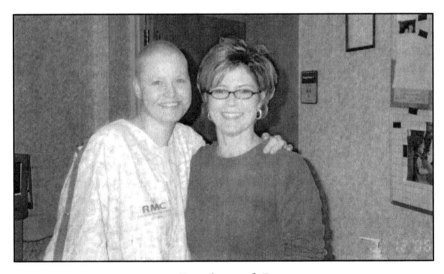

Jamie and I

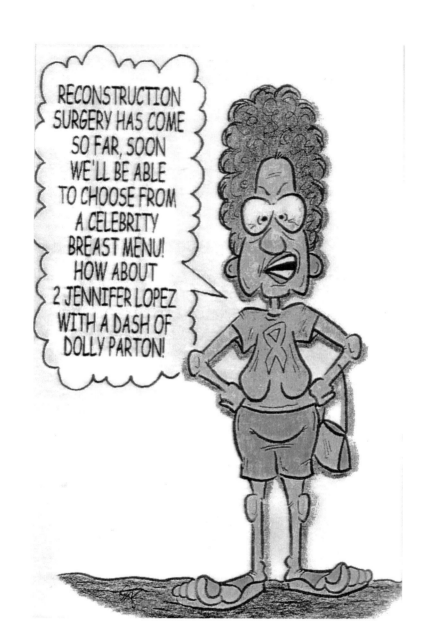

Back In the Real World

Iwas so glad to be finished with my treatment and was looking forward to having a great New Year. I was suffering from a bad case of cabin fever, so I started working with Kim at their business, Piedmont Outdoor. It felt great being around healthy people again.

May 19 was my forty-third birthday. Randa and Kim had a surprise party for me, and it was great! Many people that had supported me the past year were there. I had my reconstruction done May 25. One of the positive things that came from having breast cancer is having your insurance pay for a tummy tuck. Although the surgery lasted 10 hours, it was a success: I had a smaller waist and a new boob. I was up walking that night, which was pretty good considering I had been gutted like a fish. I stayed in the hospital three days and went home with four drain tubes…*a pain*!

I finally healed from surgery, and it was time for a nipple and tattoo. Kim took me for the procedure. When we got to the hospital, neither of us could get out of the car we were laughing so hard. She said, "They couldn't make one good body if they used both of ours, but you're going to get that nipple!"

I think the nurses must have thought we were drunk because we were laughing so much. I got my nipple, and it was the most deformed thing I had ever seen. It finally started looking normal when the swelling went down, but then it disappeared. I think it spread out when I gained weight, going from a C cup to a D cup! Oh well. Things could be worse.

Kim asked me to manage their store in the mall for Christmas. It was great to feel good and meet new people. One night at work a little boy dressed like a Christmas elf came running into the store. Did I mention we sold John Deere toy gators?

His name was Tanner, and he was two. He jumped on a toy gator, and his mom came running in behind him. They were at the mall to get Tanner's picture made. His mom forced him off the gator, and he was crying and trying to get away from her. She dragged him out of the store and down to the photographer.

A few minutes later, he came running back into the store. This happened three times. Finally, I took him down to the photographer myself. Little did I know that God was setting me up for my next job. A couple of weeks later I received a call from the director of the JCA Daycare asking if I wanted to work there. I never thought I would go through cancer to go to work teaching two and three year olds! Since Nathan and Chelsea were in school there, I agreed to take the job. I would receive a lot of benefits for working there.

Guess who came in my class within my first three weeks at work? Yep. Tanner. He remembered me, and so did his mom. They both felt really relieved. Being around the children was fun. They were all so positive and loved life. I had a great boss and coworkers and became great friends with Carmen. We had so much fun everyday. I was able to see Nathan and Chelsea at lunch each day, hear Nathan playing guitar in the worship band and see Chelsea cheer at pep rallies.

I knew God placed me there. Life was getting back to normal. My dad was in remission and so was my grandmother. I was going every three months for my checkup. My liver functions stayed high all through my chemo, so my doctor was keeping a close eye on it. I had a liver biopsy in 2009. No cancer, just a fatty liver! I could have told them that, after all those Blondies I had eaten at Applebee's. I was enjoying every day of my life. Cancer will definitely put things into proper perspective.

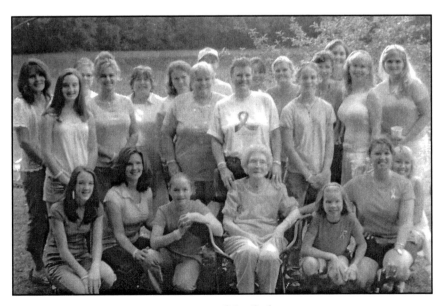

Women at my birthday party

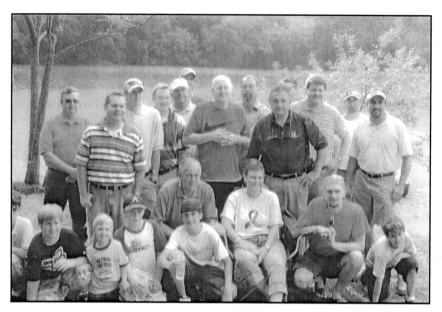

Men at my birthday party

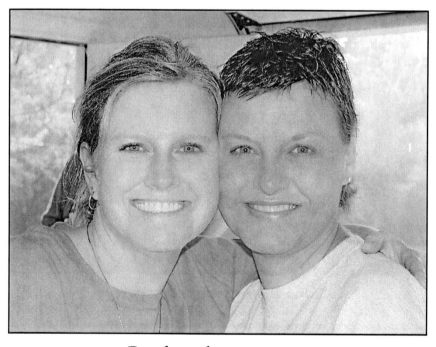

Randa and me at party

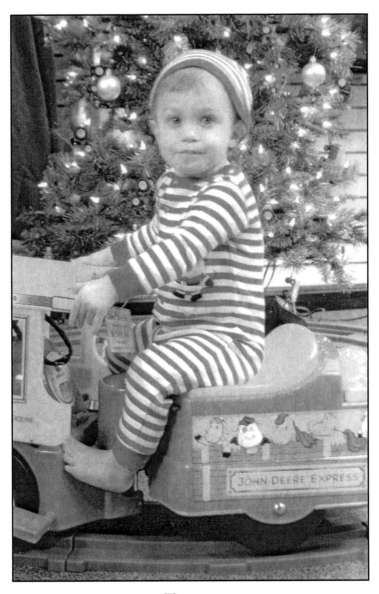

Tanner

WHEN THE SKIES ARE GRAY
AND YOU'RE FEELING BLUE,
SLAP ON A SMILE,
LET YOUR PINK SIDE
SHINE THROUGH!

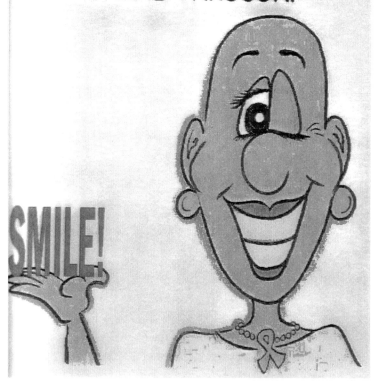

The Second Battle...Crap!

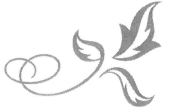

I'm going to start this chapter off by saying my new word – *Crap*.

May 29, 2011, I got a call from a friend telling me one of our high school classmates had died. I was shocked and saddened, and began calling several of my classmates, some I hadn't seen in several years.

We rented a cabin the weekend of her memorial. It was great seeing everyone again and getting caught up with everyone's lives. We laughed so much that our stomachs hurt. We named ourselves "The Ya-Ya's" and promised we'd get together every couple of months. One of my friends, Kelly, told the following story about a little boy in her class:

"The first time our paths crossed, Chase was in third grade. Visiting his classroom, I heard his very colorful language he used out loud, very loud. He was in a special class because of behavior. Fast forward a few years, and low and behold; I was informed Chase was ready for a regular classroom and I was to be his teacher. On our first day together, I was cautious, to say the least. I was quite nervous about his language. It was like inviting Honey Boo Boo's mom to be your room mom.

"However, it didn't take long for me to grow fond of Chase. I started to look forward to his morning stories. With his deep voice and slow southern drawl, he explained how you spin out on a four-wheeler. Then he would stand up and start spinning, making the motor sound. However, I started to notice he used the crap word frequently. The way he said it made it even better. It was in his low deep voice, drug out slowly. *Craap.*

Craap, I pull for Alabama.

Craap, why do you like Auburn.

Craap, I don't want hamburger for lunch.

Craap, I don't want to play dodge ball.

"My favorite was when I said, 'Get your social studies book out.' Chase yelled out 'Crap, we got to do this Crap again? We did this Crap yesterday. Why do we have to do this Crap every day?'

"The icing on the cake was when I had a meeting with his parents. It was a Friday morning, and the teacher who set up the meeting forgot to tell me. It was also Auburn / Alabama day. The best-dressed teacher would win a free day off. Needless to say, I was decked out in my orange and blue. I had my orange wig on, and I was covered in blue and orange with a tiger's tail tied around my waist. I walked into the room, and Chase's mom looked at me and said, "Crap, is that his teacher?"

We were laughing so hard our stomachs hurt; it was one of those you had to be there moments. From that time on, *Crap* became our official "Yaya's" word.

I was off for the summer and had a long list of things I wanted to get done. I had been feeling tired for about a month and didn't feel like doing anything. One day I was doing my self-exam and felt a lump. It hurt just like before. I went to the doctor, and she felt it and thought it wasn't anything to worry about. Being concerned, I immediately scheduled a mammogram. It came back abnormal, *Crap!* Did I mention I had been taking Femara medicine for five years so I wouldn't have a reccurrence?

I had a magnification mammogram. The results came in, and I had to have a biopsy my first day back at work. Two days later I got the call from Dr. Spremulli. Cancer…*Crap.*

My original oncologist, Dr. Fussell, had moved to Mississippi to take care of her parents. I really missed her, but everyone told me Dr. Spremulli was a great doctor. She did not understand my sense of humor like Dr. Fussell, but that was something I was going to work on.

Once again I had to sit my family down and tell them I had cancer, again. I felt so bad for Nathan: It was his senior year in high school, and I didn't want him worried about me. Chelsea had matured into a beautiful, caring young woman. She took care of me the first time I had cancer, and she helped me take care of my grandmother.

Curtis was the one who took it the hardest. He had a very stressful job, and the last thing he needed again was for me to be sick. I sent a message to the Yaya's that said "I have cancer again… *Crap!*"

They quickly came to support me, along with my family and co-workers. I told my boss Marla that I did great with the first cancer, and it shouldn't affect my job. Boy was I wrong.

Dr. Spremulli was very optimistic since I had caught it early; however, I would have to have another mastectomy. I decided to have reconstruction the same day as my mastectomy. I won't mention the plastic surgeon's name I met with, but the first thing he told me was I needed to lose weight. *Duh!*

He said he could help me with that: he just so happened to own a weight loss clinic. I felt that he was more concerned with my weight than my reconstruction. It would be three weeks before he and Dr. Johnson could do the surgery on the same day. It didn't take but a second to forget about reconstruction and have mastectomy, ASAP!

Surgery was scheduled that Friday, and I was happy and scared all at the same time. I was really dreading the sentinel node procedure. I found out that they use a patch to put on your breast before the procedure to help with the pain. Thank God.

The night before my surgery my friends from work, Kim, Randa,and Bob and I went to a local restaurant to have a going away party for my boob, complete with a boob cake and pink cigars. People could not believe we were laughing and celebrating having breast cancer, but I learned through the first cancer that when you laugh, you are winning.

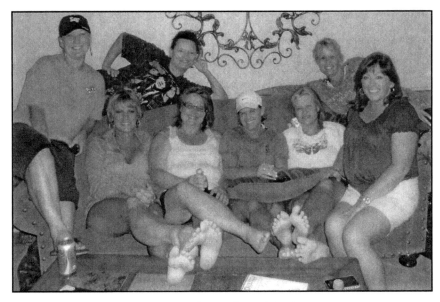

YaYa Reunion 2011

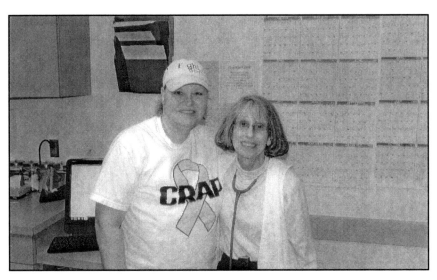

Dr. Spremulli and I

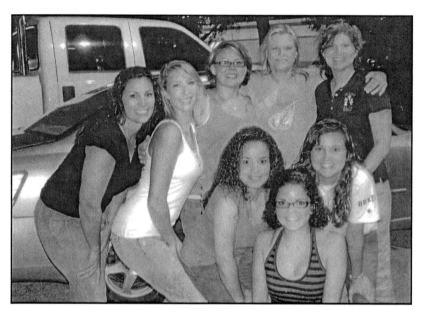

JCCDC friends

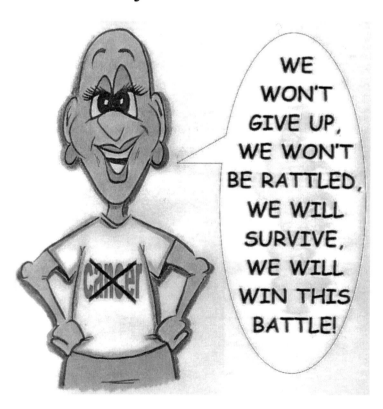

Surgery Day

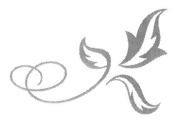

Everything went according to plan. It was weird having an IV in my left arm; for five years they could not do anything on my left side. Dr. Johnson came in with the good news that it had not moved to my lymph nodes. I was really drugged out after surgery as my friends started coming by the hospital. Becky brought me a box so we could have a memorial service for my boob at the beach. Belinda came and brought me a shirt that had the breast cancer symbol with the word CRAP written across it. It was a very funny moment and I didn't realize at the time how important that shirt would become.

Ya-Ya Beach Trip

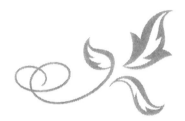

We decided we'd go to the beach before my chemo treatments were to start. Our former high school teacher, Kay Kisor, let us stay at her beautiful condo at Orange Beach. There were ten of us that made the trip, and we had a blast!

The weather was beautiful. I pulled the cancer card, and we went on a catamaran ride and saw dolphins everywhere. Everyone had a crap shirt, and that's what we wore to have our picture made. After we made pictures, we went to The Wharf where there is a huge Ferris wheel and many shops and restaurants.

All night people would ask us what crap meant, and we would say it means cancer is *crap*! Nobody got it until we got to the Ferris wheel, and we walked up to a guy who worked there that said, "I know what that means."

His name was Michael, and his aunt had just been diagnosed with breast cancer. He let us ride for free, but one of my friends, Dana, was terrified of Ferris wheels and didn't want to ride. I pulled the cancer card on her, and she rode it, twice. It was a great night. The last night we were there we went down to the beach and sat around my boob box and celebrated its life with me. We were going to bury it in the sand, but I decided I wanted to bring it home and remember the great trip we had. Reality set in when I got home. I started chemo in two weeks. *Crap.*

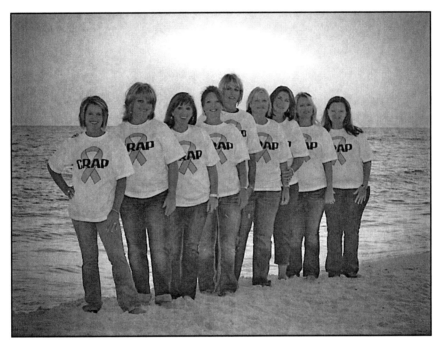

Yaya's In CRAP shirt

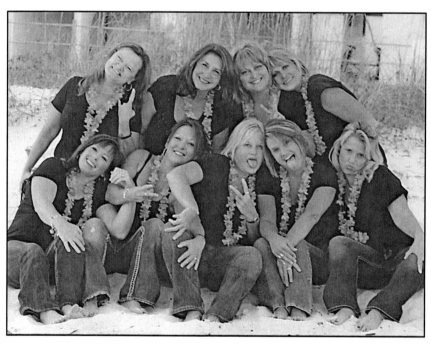

Yaya's being goofy

The Port From Hell

Dr. Johnson was out of town when I called to set an appointment to have my port put in. Since my chemo was starting in a few days, I couldn't wait for him to get back into town. The nurse said another doctor - who will remain nameless - could put the port in the next day. I readily agreed. It was a simple procedure. What could go wrong, right?

The doctor did the procedure at the surgery room at her office. I went for my first chemo, and I had sludge in my port. It took forever for the nurse to get it to flush. That was the beginning of the slippery slope of what was to happen in my life with cancer number two.

I was feeling like I had cancer for the first time, again. I officially had chemo brain once again, and nothing was going like the first time. I had a lot of nausea.

I wanted life to remain as normal as possible, so even though I felt sick, Kim and I took Chelsea and Calley to see the movie "The Help." It only made me mad at white people. The movie reminded me of a black lady who helped my Grandmother Bragg when I was little named Viola. I loved her so much.

WE VE GOT FAITH
IN OUR HEARTS
AND GOD ON OUR SIDE.
LET'S WAVE OUR
PINK RIBBONS,
FOR WE WILL
SURVIVE!

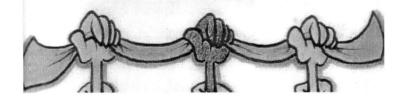

MRSA and CRAP

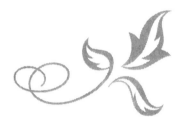

I woke up Monday morning with what looked like an ant bite on my neck. It was very red and painful to the touch. I worked all week feeling very tired and sick at my stomach, but when I woke up Friday morning, I had a fever, and my neck was swollen all the way down to the port. I went to the surgeon who put the port in, and she said it looked infected, sent me home with strong antibiotics, and told me if I was no better on Monday, she might have to remove the port. I went home and went to sleep.

When I woke up two hours later, my fever was up to one-hundred and three degrees, and I was in intense pain. Becky carried me to Dr. Spremulli who said it was staph infection. She took a culture and sent me right to the hospital. One of the perks of being a chemo patient is that you get a "fast pass" into the emergency room. No sitting in the waiting room; the nurse carries you immediately back.

For the first time after having cancer, I was very scared. I had an awful night with lots of pain and a high fever. Randa stayed with me and kept the nurses on their toes. The next morning Dr. Johnson came in and said he was removing the port. *Thank God!* I felt so much better just having it removed. The nurse came in and told me it was MRSA, a much more difficult to treat type of staph infection.

Kelly came to the hospital determined to have the doctor put a feeding tube in me so she could fill me up with carrot juice. *Not happening!* They already had me on the right antibiotics for MRSA. I had a big hole in my chest that looked horrible and a long road to recover from infection, and I'd have to begin seeing an infectious disease doctor. The doctor came in and said the infection was not in my blood, that I could go home and would not have to go with a PICC line, and that I could take meds by mouth. Randa and Becky were in the room; we all were very happy.

Be still and you hear it,

It's the sound of your spirit,

It will guide you

Don't fear it,

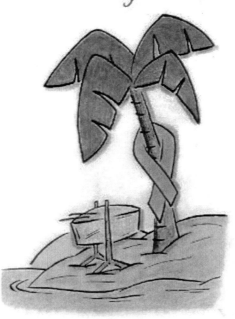

Survival's your fate,

Rejoice as you near it!

God Shows Up

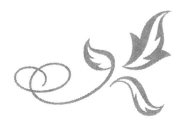

Ihad been so sick all week that I couldn't eat, but after the good news, I wanted a hamburger and fries. I was enjoying the food when a social worker from the hospital came in and said I could not leave the hospital until they knew I could get my meds, which would cost $3,894.78! I would have to pay for them up front, and the insurance would reimburse me eighty percent.

My happiness turned to nausea really fast. I told her I did not have that much money. She asked if I had $800 to cover the twenty percent. I said crap, I didn't have $20! I told her to call Curtis.

Randa was crying. I assured her it was all right, I would just stay in the hospital. Randa then informed me that I did have $800.

Without my knowing it, my family and friends had sold over one-hundred crap shirts. I started to cry. I could not believe it, and I was so humbled and thankful for Randa and my friends.

I was still getting over the emotion from the t-shirt sales when the same social worker walked in and handed me a check for $3,894; the auxiliary at the hospital hold fund raisers all year so they can help people. She said for me to bring the check from the insurance company back to the hospital when we received it. How great is our God!

I was released from the hospital, got my medicine, and was finally at home. It felt so good to be there with no IV attached to me. I slept so well. The next day my buddies from work brought me lunch and a check. I was out of sick days, but they pooled and given me theirs. What awesome friends I have! I was having a great day when Kelly showed up with her ninja blender and a case of carrots. She was determined I was going to drink carrot juice. Becky came over to help with the blending, and everything in the kitchen was turning orange. I gave in and drank a full glass…*not happening.* I appreciated her concern about my health, but that was not what I was going to do. I thought I'd just purchase several bottles of ranch dressing for the kids to eat with the carrots.

Kayron came up from Tuscaloosa and brought a comedy to watch. It was great laughing again. JCA had a football game that night, and I wanted to go see Chelsea cheer. I'd missed much since I'd been sick. I made it to halftime but had to leave then because I was very tired. It was great getting to see everyone and being outdoors. We take so much for granted when we are well.

I went for my first visit to the doctor since I got out of the hospital. Dr. Spremulli said it looked as though the surgeon had left part of the tube in my neck when he took my port out. *What?*

She ordered an ultrasound on my neck. They checked my counts, and since they were good, I could have chemo. I had no port so I was forced to do chemo with an IV. *Crap.* Thank God the nurse found a vein the first time she tried. Of course, that vein could never be used again. *I hate chemo.*

I found a recliner close to the snacks and fridge and started my dose of poison. After the chemo was over, I went to the hospital for my ultrasound. They found a blood clot in my jugular vein. You have *got* to be kidding. I had to go back to the doctor's office to be told that I'd have to do injections in my stomach twice a day until finished with chemo. I hate needles. *Crap.*

I finally got home and learned the shots would cost $4,000 a month. *Here we go again.* I couldn't wait to see how God would work that out. I called Kay, Dr. Spremulli's nurse, and told her I couldn't get the shots. She told me to come in, fill out an application, and she would send it to a pharmaceutical company. In the meantime, Randa and my friends were busy selling shirts. I had so many people going the second mile for me. I'm so blessed. It took a couple of days, but I discovered the pharmaceutical company would send me three months of shots! *Thank God!*

One week after getting out of the hospital, I noticed my hair had begun to come out, and this time I was on it. I did not want to wait until it was coming out by the handfuls, so I called Randa and Bob and told them it was time. They came over with the dog clippers. Becky had already cut it off as short as she could with the scissors. I thought I would be a little bit creative this time, so I told Bob to make me a Mohawk. That style lasted until Curtis got home and told me that it had to go. Party pooper!

My grandmother had been in the nursing home for about a year. I had always promised her I would take care of her. She had taken care of me my whole life, and we were very close. When she became unable to live by herself, she and my dad decided it would be best that she go into the nursing home. The fact that I was not able to take care of her was very hard for me.

She wasn't happy at first, but she got into a private room, and Randa fixed it up really nice for her. She was very worried about me and my health, and was always thinking about her family.

One day she began acting differently. She wouldn't eat, and she was talking incoherently. They took her to the hospital to be evaluated where it was discovered she had early dementia. It happened so suddenly. I refused to believe that my Grandmother would forget who I was. I started praying and asked God to bring her mind back. I fully believed He would. I had to start going to a wound doctor for my chest where the port was infected. I saw Nan, a lady from church and told her about Grandmother. She prayed with me for her each time I went to the doctor.

Chelsea's sixteenth birthday was approaching and I was determined to throw her a party. Randa took me to Oxford to get party supplies, and my friend Jane gave me lots of stuff she had left over from her daughter's party. Everything was coming together. Everyone pitched in and helped decorate, and it looked great! I couldn't believe my baby was sixteen. She grew up way too fast.

The party was so much fun. Becky, Kelly, and I did karaoke, and Kelly came complete with a tambourine. I did "The Wop" with Chelsea. I was so tired, but so happy to be there. Belinda brought in the crap shirts and everyone at the party got one. I was very humbled.

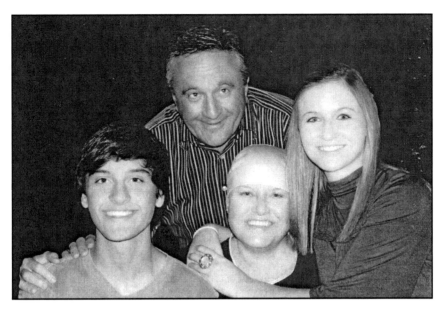

Family at Chelsea's Party

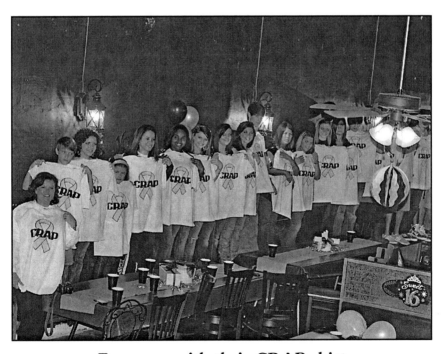

Everyone with their CRAP shirt

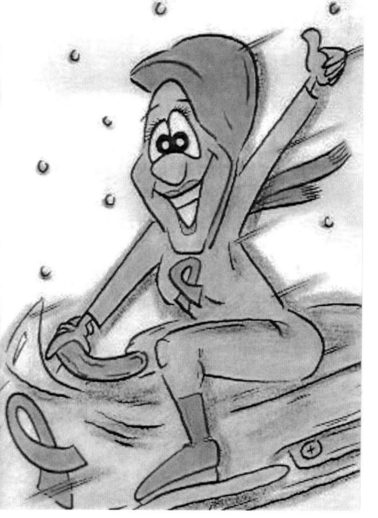

I Finally Get A Jeep

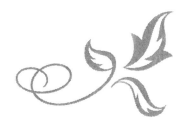

As I mentioned before, I had always wanted a jeep. Curt would say, "Not practical". I told him during my first cancer I wanted a jeep before I died. Well…I think after the MRSA and blood clot he was concerned that I might not make it, so he called one morning and told me to go pick up the 2010 jeep wrangler I had been asking for! *Yes!* I don't recommend getting one the way I had to, but I love it.

I woke up feeling really bad, so I went to the doctor, who said my counts were down more than they had ever been. I was staying nauseated all the time. She put me under house arrest, and I'd have to wear a mask when I went out.

Chelsea was chosen for the Homecoming Court at school. I could not miss that, I thought. *I hate cancer.*

I took the top off the jeep and rode down every country road I could find. The leaves had begun to change, and it was beautiful. I went to the pep rally and all the people from work and the children had on pink do-rags. *Very cool*. It was rainy and cold, but I was determined I wasn't missing the football game. Chelsea looked beautiful, and Curtis didn't look bad either.

I got a call from the nursing home at the end of the game; Grandmother had come back to herself and was asking for us! We were all at the game, so we rushed to see her. It was a miracle. She was eating when we got there, and I'd never been so happy to see her. We take people in our lives for granted so much. We never know how long we are going to have the people we love here on earth.

It was November 1. I couldn't believe how fast time was going by. I love the holidays. I always start in November listening to Christmas music and putting up decorations. After all I have been through; no one has to tell me to be thankful.

During the first cancer, I learned how short life can be and how to appreciate every day as a gift. Now, I appreciate every minute I'm not sitting in the chemo room, in the hospital, or nauseated.

It was time to have my port put back in. I will never say again that it is a simple procedure. Dr. Johnson would be putting it in this time. Everything went great. I was supposed to have chemo right immediately afterward, but Dr. S said I could wait a couple of days. They did my lab work, and I told the doctor that this nausea was not from chemo. She said it might be my gallbladder. *Seriously?*

My liver counts came back higher than ever, so she wanted me to see my gastrologist and have tests run. They checked my gallbladder function and did an ultrasound. Yep. It was my gallbladder. I couldn't believe it, there was a blockage in the duct going from my gallbladder to my liver. I'd have to have surgery after my next chemo.

Let's review:

1. I find out I have cancer, *again.*
2. I have a mastectomy, *again.*
3. I get MRSA staff infection from my port.
4. They find a blood clot in my jugular vein.
5. My counts are low, I miss chemo and I get put under house arrest.
6. I have to have gallbladder surgery.
7. Three hospital stays.

Yes! I was thankful to be alive that Thanksgiving. I had the surgery right before Thanksgiving, and I was amazed at how much better I felt. Just in time to enjoy all the food! Grandmother had always helped me decorate our Christmas tree, so I went to the nursing home and brought her to the house to watch. She wasn't able to get around very well, but I was so grateful she was with me and back to herself again. Looking around at my family and all we had been through the past year, I was so blessed and thankful for all I had.

I arrived at chemo to see all my nurses in my Team Venecia Christmas shirts that Randa designed and sold for me. *Very cool.* Of course, I had to get a picture, and we all laugh every time we see it. The man sitting next to me was sound asleep, and the nurses pushed his chair out of the way so they could all get in the picture. The snack basket was filled with extra candy and treats people had brought for me and my fellow chemo-ers. I was all over that. My nurse was excited to see the homemade candy tray Randa and Bob made for them. (They make the best fudge I have ever eaten.) I was so thankful my nausea had gone away, even if it meant losing my gallbladder. Well, it was time to put in a Madea movie and laugh while the poison was hopefully killing the cancer cells in my body.

I may have mentioned this before, but Christmas is my favorite time of year. Everyone seems to be more caring and thankful that time of year. I know for myself, I am thankful every time God allows me to wake up and have another day to live. I love watching old Christmas movies with Nathan and Chelsea and drinking hot chocolate. "The Year without a Santa Claus" is my favorite.

Chelsea had a lead role in the Christmas play at school. They performed "It's a Wonderful Life," and she did a great job. Nathan played the guitar. I am amazed how talented she and Nathan are; I think they got it from their dad, but I'll take the credit for their sense of humor.

I had chemo the week before Christmas, so I was very tired but very thankful that my family was all there with me. Even though Nathan was 17 and Chelsea 16, I still loved to see their faces on Christmas morning when they discovered what Santa brought. Traditionally, we go to my parents' house for Christmas breakfast. Grandmother was not able to be there that year. She was not able to get out of bed and sit up for a long length of time, and I missed her very much. It was the first time she has not been there with us.

After opening presents at my parents, we went to the nursing home and spent time with her. I was thankful for her caretakers at the nursing home. They took very good care of her. After Christmas, Becky, Belinda, Kayron, Kelly, Sharon and I went to my parents' home in Tennessee for a few days. We ate and shopped until we dropped. After arriving home on New Year's Eve, Curtis and I watched the ball drop and I hit the hay. I was very tired, but very excited to see what 2012 had in store for me. Dr. Johnson told me when I had my first cancer that it would be the worst year of my life. Actually, the past year had been the worst as far as my health was concerned. My New Year's resolution was to enjoy everyday that God gave me and never take anyone in my life for granted.

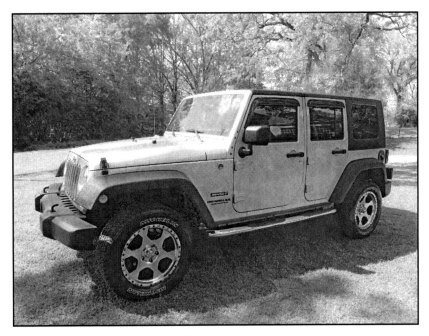

My Jeep

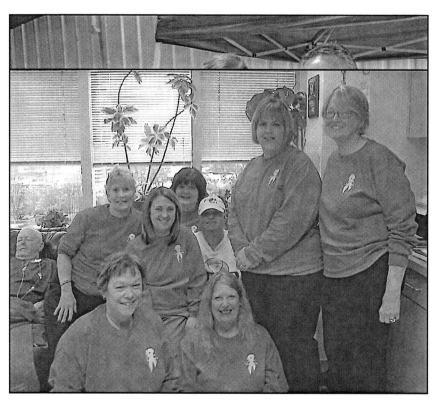

My nurses and me

My Last Chemo Treatment...Again!

January 18, 2012. My last chemo treatment. I can proudly say I made it through every treatment without watching "The Price Is Right." Major accomplishment.

I am thankful I am not a casualty in this war, but I will forever have the scars from it. As I looked around the chemo room, I saw all the chairs filled by people from all walks of life, some of them close to the end of their life; survivor's guilt overcame me. I felt so blessed to be at the end of my second battle with this awful disease. Although there had been many times I had felt that I wouldn't survive, I had pulled through. I know there is a reason God allowed me to endure all this, and my prayer for 2012 was to find my purpose and not waste one day of the rest of my life.

As I watched the last of the poison go through my IV, I realized all I had done was reflect over the past six month, and pray for my fellow cancer warriors. I thought about my family and friends who stood beside me, and how much they had done for me. I am blessed! As the nurse flushed my port and that awful taste came to my mouth, I was ready to run, but I felt a terrible sadness for the people who would be back the next week.

Two weeks had passed since my last chemo treatment. I still had to take the lovenox injections until my port was taken out, followed by a bone scan and a pet scan. It took a couple of days for me to get results from the doctor.

Finally, the call came. All clear! Thank God! Then I could call Dr. Johnson to arrange to have my port taken out and meet with Dr. Fix about my new boob.

I was back in an all-too-familiar place, the outpatient surgery unit at the hospital. Dr. Johnson came in and said he could take out my port without putting me to sleep. *Crap.* I am one crazy tough person. After all I had been through, that wasn't that bad. I had no recovery time. I just jumped off the table, put my clothes on and went home. No more injections.

My Second New Boob...Not!

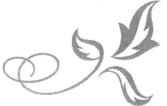

When my port finally healed, I met with Dr. Fix about my reconstruction. He was concerned about me having a blood clot and gave me two different options: Have an IGAP-Inferior gluteal artery perforator flap - take fat from my butt - or get an implant. My choice was to take half of my left breast, which is actually my belly and a size larger than it was when I had it put on, and put it on my right side. Unfortunately, that was not an option.

I did not want an implant. Who doesn't want some fat removed from their butt? It would be a ten to twelve hour surgery, and with any surgery there was a chance of getting a blood clot, so Dr. Fix wanted me to have extensive blood work done. Dee, Dr. Fix assistant, called and said my liver counts were very high and so was my clotting level. Dr. Fix said he would not want to put me to sleep until Dr. Hixon could check my liver and then come back and have labs done again in three months. Dr. Hixon sent me for a scan of my liver. Still just a fatty liver. Dr. Hixon called and told Dr. Fix it would acceptable for me to have the surgery. I really wasn't in a hurry to have surgery. Getting a new boob was not worth taking a chance of a blood clot developing in my heart. Dr. Fix wanted to wait three months at what time he would redo blood work.

My Grandmother, My Angel

We had just celebrated grandmother's eighty-seventh birthday. She was almost completely bed ridden by then. Since I was finished with chemo; I could spend more time with her. Because it was dangerous for me to be around sickness, I was unable to visit her for a week when the nursing home had a virus outbreak.

It was so difficult watching someone I love so much come to the end of her life, and I felt so helpless. I tried to get there in time to feed her lunch because I could always get her to eat more than the aide. She always told me if she ever reached the point at which she couldn't talk, to make sure she had cornbread and milk. Dutifully, I told the therapist, who made sure she had cornbread every day. I would sit there and we'd talk and laughed about all the crazy things we had done over the years. I've always had her undivided attention.

When I was little, we would talk on the phone for hours, just like best friends. She lived across from the elementary school I attended, and some mornings she would call me and say, "Do you feel like going to school today?"

Of course I would say "no!" I'd tell the teacher I was sick, and they would call her, and she would walk to the school and check me out, and we would play the rest of the day. We would color; sing songs, and watch her "story" "The Young and the Restless." She would fix my favorites for lunch: fried chicken, creamed potatoes, slaw, and of course, a chocolate pudding. After lunch we would go out to play ball or do anything I wanted to do. She used to love a cold Dr. Pepper in a bottle. We would sit on the porch and drink one after we played awhile.

She would tell me stories about when she was young, like picking cotton, walking across the frozen creek in the winter to get to school and all the mischievous things she and her siblings did. I know who I inherited that from. When I was twenty-two, I had moved ninety miles away to Birmingham. I would talk to her every day on the phone, and when I would come home, she'd make me fried chicken, biscuits, and a strawberry cake to carry back with me. She didn't know it, but sometimes those meals and frosted flakes were all I had to eat.

No one was happier than my grandmother when I moved back home two years later. She worried all the time. I met Curtis a year later, and we were married June 23, 1990. Nathan was born three years later, and I quit work to be home with him. Grandmother came over every day and spent time with Nathan and me. It was as if she was revived having a baby to take care of. Eighteen months later Chelsea was born. She became grandmother's little Jewel. (Jewel was grandmother's little girl who died at only nine months old with pneumonia.)

I was so happy to know my children would have her in their lives. She would play with them, watch Barney, Blues

Clues and her favorite, Little Bear, every day with them. The summer after Chelsea was born; the house we were renting sold forcing us to move. We had already found a house to buy but, it was going to be a few months before we could move in. Grandmother insisted that we stay with her.

Her house was small and became even smaller when two more adults, two children, and one puppy moved in, but she couldn't have been happier. Chelsea learned to walk at her house. I have many great memories of that time. When Nathan and Chelsea were seven and five years old, I decided to home school them using videos from Pensacola Christian School. I loved being with them all the time. Grandmother stayed with us through the winter, and she would sit and watch while both of them did their schoolwork. She said she was learning things as well.

I remember the day she said she needed to go back to her house. I told her she didn't have to go, but she insisted. We packed her belongings, and I took her home. When I got home, I broke down and cried. Chelsea said; "Go get her Mom" so off I went back to her house. She had just finished putting her clothes up, and I said, "Let's go." We both started crying, and I repacked her things and brought her back to our house. She stayed with us a lot until I was diagnosed with cancer the first time. When it reached the point that she could no longer live by herself, she and Daddy decided it would be best for her to go into the nursing home. She had been there fourteen months, when on March 22, Randa called and said the nurse called and said Grandmother was not doing well.

Randa, Chelsea, and I got there to find her soaking wet from sweating and breathing very hard. We told them to call the hospice nurse to come check her. She came and said

Grandmother was in the final stages before death. The nurse started giving her morphine to keep her from having to work so hard to breathe. Daddy and Mother were at their home in Tennessee. I called him and let him talk to the nurse. He said he would be there in the morning.

I stayed with her all night. We had to change her bed three times because she was sweating so much. The nurse said her body was working so hard to live. I told her we would be all right and that she had done a great job of taking care of us and that she needed to go rest. That was the hardest thing I've ever said. I didn't want her to suffer anymore, but I couldn't imagine my life without her.

Daddy and Mother arrived the next morning, and the people from hospice were there. They were so kind, bringing food and coffee for us and praying with us. All of us were there with her throughout the day. I was lying on the bed beside her. The nurse said she could hear me, so I kept telling her I loved her and I would see her again. She went to Heaven at 4 p.m. The aides came in to bathe her, and I asked if I could do it. She always told me I gave her the best bath. I couldn't keep the tears wiped off fast enough. I stayed with her until the man from the funeral home came to get her. As he carried her away, I felt like my heart was breaking, but then I realized she was now my angel. At her funeral we played the song *My Angel* by Kellie Picker as a tribute to her.

I will see you again; *Rest in peace Grandmother, I love you.*

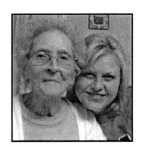

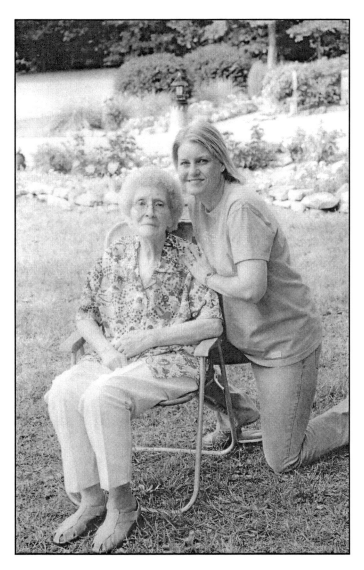

Look to your heart
and your strength
will astound you,
Your prayers will
be answered
and peace will
surround you,
You must dry your eyes
for the future awaits,
With patience and courage
survival's your fate

Life Goes On

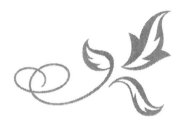

Curtis and I took Nathan and Chelsea to Gulf Shores for their spring break. I was still grieving over grandmother, but I had been looking forward to spending time with the family. After the last seven months of sickness and chemo, I was glad to feel like going somewhere. Every time I go to the beach I am amazed at Gods creation and how big the ocean is. We went to the Wharf. I wanted the family to meet Michael. We rode the Ferris wheel three times. It seemed as though just the day before I was with the Ya-Yas there, and Dana was scared to death! Each night I sat on the balcony and thanked God for letting me live, and instead of me telling Him what I was going to do, I asked Him to tell me what He wanted me to do. A person doesn't live through cancer twice and not have a purpose for being on the earth. I knew I wanted to do something to help people. After seeing how great the people from hospice were, I thought maybe I should try to work with them. Marla and everybody at work had been so good to me; my plan was if God didn't open another door was to have reconstruction and go back to JCCDC in August.

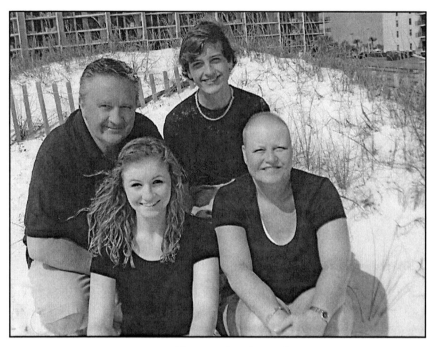

Family at the beach

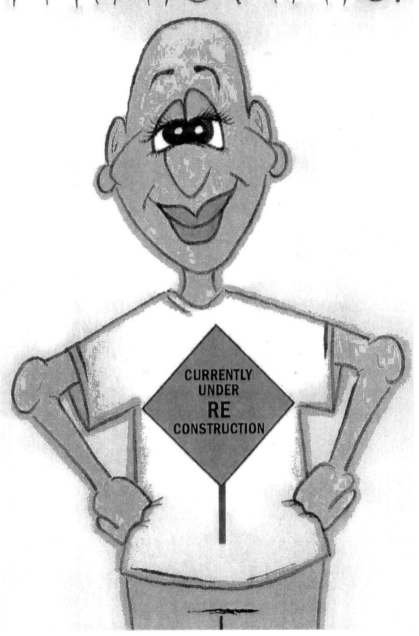

Birthday...Party...Graduation...Party... Reconstruction...Not Happening

It was May. Wow, how time had flown by! That year at the Relay for Life, there were forty of my friends wearing their crap shirts, all coming to walk with me. That was a great night! My birthday had arrived again, and I was so happy to be celebrating another year here on this earth. Randa had a party for me at the Solid Rock Café. All my friends showed up, and we had a great night complete, with karaoke and Kelly with her tambourine.

Some of the mothers and I were planning a party for graduation. I couldn't believe Nathan would be graduating. I remember the first time I had cancer he was finishing his sixth grade year and I had asked God to please let me live to raise him and Chelsea. And now, two cancers and six years later, he was graduating. Thank you, God, for letting me be here.

I loved all the students and teachers at JCA: they had been so supportive of me. The party was a success but bitter sweet for us parents. Nathan's graduation was the next night, and I was, and am, so proud of him. Thanks to my friend Patty Carroll, he got a job with the City of Jacksonville.

It was time to go back to Dr. Fix and have my lab taken. He said if numbers were still high, it would be too dangerous to put me to sleep for reconstruction. I asked if he could liposuction some of the fat out of my remaining breast so I wouldn't look so bad. He said he could. When results came back, there would be no reconstruction for me just then. In fact, the numbers were still so high the doctor wouldn't do anything to me. *Crap!*

I didn't know when I would look normal again. My prosthetic breast was heavy and very uncomfortable, leaving no doubt in my mind that a man invented it. Consequently, most of the time I would just wear a comfortable sports bra and go around with only one boob.

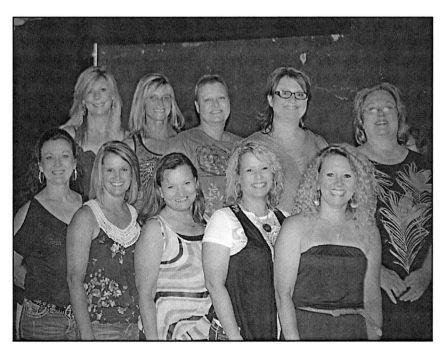

Friends at my birthday party

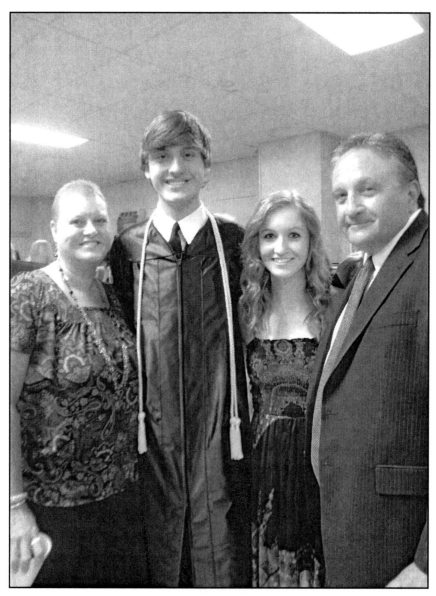

Nathan's Graduation

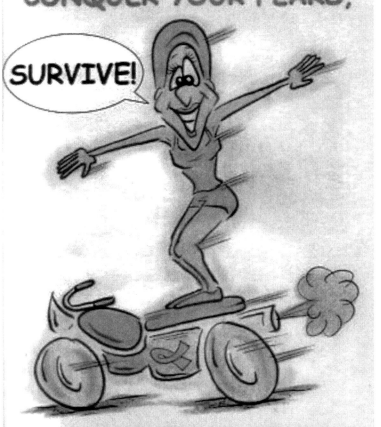

I Find My Purpose, And My Third Tumor

I was still waiting for God to tell me why I was alive and what He wanted me to do, so I prayed and went back to work at JCCDC. After working two weeks, I was in the bathroom changing a diaper when I heard God say, "I want you to write and speak."

I know one could think since I was changing diapers the idea of writing and speaking might have seemed like something great to do. Let me enlighten you a bit. In high school I had paid someone to write my book reports, and my counselor had told me I was not college material. My highest accomplishment had been receiving the award for most mischievous. I don't like to read books, and I really destroy the English language. I was much more comfortable changing diapers than even thinking about writing and speaking. I don't know how many of you have heard God speak, but I have, and I knew what I was supposed to do.

Leaving the baby with a coworker, I went straight into Marla's office and turned in my notice. I have heard people say that God doesn't call the equipped; He equips the called. I was hoping this to be true because I could neither write nor speak; It wasn't any time until the phone began ringing with people asking me to come speak at their church or women's group, and I began writing. I was amazed at how easy it was for me: I had been keeping journals since my first cancer.

That very week I felt a knot on my chest wall near my mastectomy scar. I went to Dr Spremulli who wanted Dr. Johnson to biopsy it. I didn't tell anyone about it and went alone to Dr. Johnson for a sonogram.

Like twice before, I asked if the lump was fluid filled. The response, "NO". *I could not believe this was happening.* Dr. Johnson, hoping it was a fatty tumor, said he could biopsy it right then, and I readily agreed.

After the procedure, I called Curtis and said, Well, I've just had a biopsy." He was unhappy and shocked all at the same time. On the drive home, I realized why God didn't allow me to have the reconstruction surgery: If I had gotten another breast, I would not have been able to feel the knot on my chest. I thanked God for taking care of me once again.

October is breast cancer awareness month, and Becky had a great idea of celebrating breast cancer survivors at The Solid Rock Café in Piedmont. She called it "The Solid Rock goes pink." I thought it was a great idea. Although we had only two weeks to coordinate the event, I knew that it would all come together with Becky and Randa at the helm. I called Eddie Burkhalter, who was a writer for The Piedmont Journal. He met with Becky, Randa, and me and we told him about the event and I shared my story with him. He was very excited and accommodating with my story and the plans. I did not mention to him about my latest discovery; I did not want to tell anyone until I heard from my biopsy.

September 28, Kay called with the news. It was cancer. *Crap!* It was on my chest wall. I knew God knew this was going to happen, and I remembered what He had told me to do, so I would do what I had to in order to battle it again. I would write and go anywhere invited to speak. I had already spoken twice and had seven more speaking engagements lined up in October. We had the celebration at The Solid Rock October 6. It was a huge success with more than two-hundred people attending. When the newspaper came out, I started getting more invitations to speak, including one to speak to the teen girls at a women's conference.

I love seeing how God orchestrates my life. While Randa and I were sitting at my crap table, the key note speaker came up to me and started talking. I told her my story and how God told me to write and speak. I told her I didn't know anything about getting a book published. She smiled and said, "I used to work at Lifeway." For those not familiar with Lifeway, the company is one of the biggest Christian publishing companies on the planet! She wrote down the name of the person I would need to talk to about publishing my book.

Crap and ZTA

I contacted my pastor about October being Breast Cancer Awareness month and asked if he would show my crap shirt to the church and say something about breast cancer. Of course he agreed, and I invited several of my family and friends to church, requesting that they wear their crap shirts.

On the way home, I noticed that ZTA girls at JSU were putting up pink ribbons all over Jacksonville, an annual event they do for breast cancer awareness. Becky was with me, and when we passed the college, I saw a group of ZTA's standing close to the road, so I quickly whipped my jeep in, scaring Becky to death. Sporting our crap shirts, we jumped out, and I asked them to come over and talk. I told them I appreciated what they were doing and relayed my story. I said, "You need to hook me up with your president so I can come speak at a ZTA meeting." One of the girls spoke up and said, "My name is Katie, and I'm the president!" *Okay Dokey! How cool is that?* Out of seventy-five ZTA girls I almost ran over the president! She said they had a meeting the following Tuesday at 8 p.m., and I told her I would be there. I gave them all a crap emblem for their car window, and we took off. That is how God orchestrates my life. I tell people I am an "unofficial" ZTA now and I have seventy-five little "sisters".

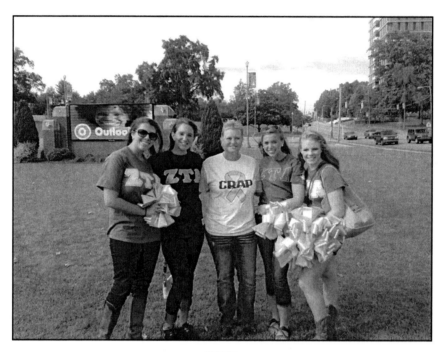

ZTA

My Second Trip to the Nuclear Spa

My first visit with Dr. Trupp was October 9. When I got off the elevator, guess what was on the TV? "The Price is Right!" *OMG!* After I checked in I told the receptionist Pam about my experience with that show, and she allowed me to go on back to the other waiting area. As I was walking by, I shot the TV with my make believe gun.

I started radiation October 29. I would have to have forty treatments. It was good seeing Jamie and Sandy, friends that had worked at the nuclear spa when I went in 2006. They were the women who pushed the button to zap me. That time the entire right side of my chest would be treated. That was going to leave a mark!

Radiation was making me feel tired, but I still spoke six times in November. I am so amazed how God opened doors for me.

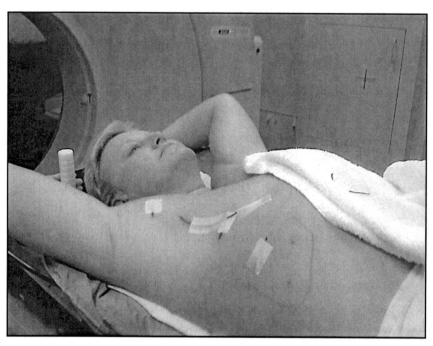

Starting my 2nd radiation

Crap Worldwide

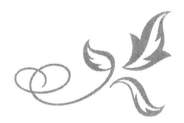

Chelsea was going to an Auburn football game with friends Kim and Calley. I thought it would be fun to have her take my crap shirt to the ballgame and have my friend Trent, a photojournalist at a local newspaper, take her photo while in the stands. The picture was great, and it gave me the idea to tell people to take their picture with my shirt wherever they journeyed. I told my friends that *crap* was going worldwide, and that is what happened.

People started posting pictures on my Facebook page from Afghanistan, Paris, London, Philippines, and places in the U.S. like Disney World, Indiana, New York, Minnesota, Las Vegas, Florida, Savannah and North Carolina. I had pictures of my friends with country singer Jamey Johnson, Go Radio, the Florida State cheerleaders, the Bear Bryant and Nick Saban statue and, of course the Coaches Trophy in Tuscaloosa. It made me smile to see the thoughtfulness of people.

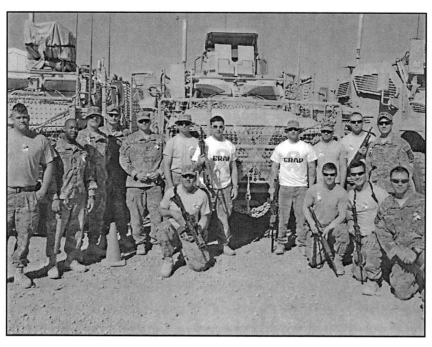

The 1 167th Infantry in Afghanistan

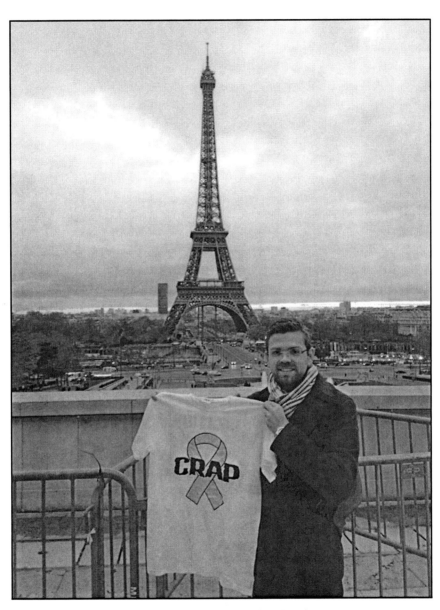

Mitchell Rogers in Paris

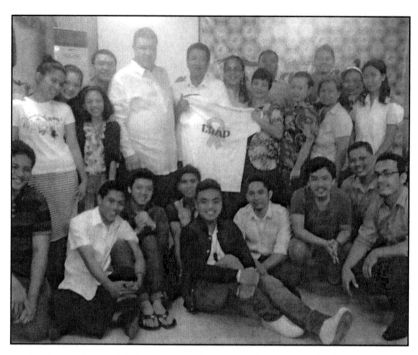

Edward and Florence Isidoro in the Philippines

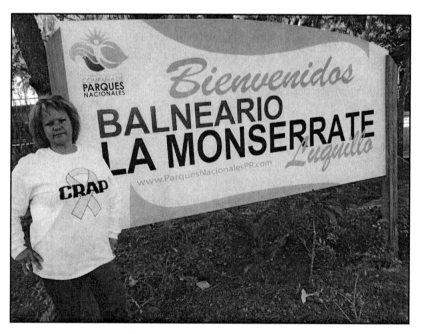

Maria Crespo in Puerto Rico

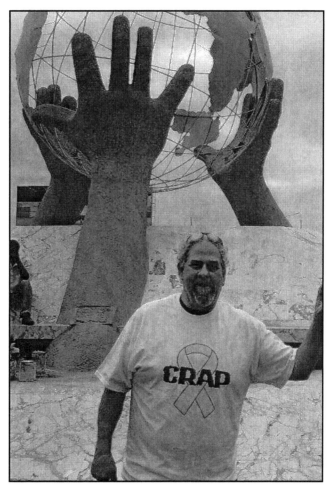

David Gunter in Port au Prince Haiti

My Talk

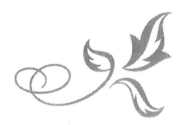

When I started pondering what God wanted me to speak about, I knew it was not going to be all about me. I wanted people who heard me to think about their own lives and leave changed. I knew there were two things I would carry every time I spoke: my green chair and a picture of my grandmother and me. I miss her so much, and I know if she was still here and able, she would go with me when I spoke. When I speak now, I sit in my green chair with my grandmother's picture beside me. Sometimes I play the songs *This Ain't Nothing* by Craig Morgan, *If Today Was Your Last Day* by Nickel back or *Beautiful Day* by U2. Although they all have a powerful meaning, I especially like the song *Beautiful Day* because after you go through cancer, no matter what day it is or what the weather is doing, it is always a beautiful day. The song also reminds me of Nathan when he was one-and-a-half years old.

We had gone to eat lunch with Grandmother. It was a gloomy day: The sun was hidden behind clouds, and it was sprinkling rain. As I took Nathan out of the car, he looked up at the sky with a big smile on his face and said, "Mommy, it is a beautiful day!" I understand what he meant now.

I tell about Pastor Kent and the do-rag, my chair and the cloud-to-ground lighting experience. I tell the audience of Randa and my friends selling crap shirts and how I couldn't have made it without God and my friends and family going the second mile for me. I tell people to look for God encounters everyday: opportuntunities to go that extra mile, or to respond positively with a smile when asked how you are doing. People are not used to that. There is a purpose for every person God sends into your life. Sometimes one word can give someone a breakthrough. Are you one of those people who hate their job, or won't be happy until Friday when you get off work or during the holidays or vacation? This is for you:

Written by Jason Lehman, a teenage boy wise beyond his years.

Present Tense

It was spring, but it was summer I wanted,
the warm days, and the great outdoors.
It was summer, but it was fall I wanted,
the colorful leaves, and the cool, dry air.
It was fall, but it was winter I wanted,
the beautiful snow, and the joy of the holiday season.
It was winter, but it was spring I wanted,
the warmth and the blossoming of nature.
I was a child, but it was adulthood I wanted,
the freedom and respect.
I was 20, but it was 30 I wanted,
to be mature, and sophisticated.

I was middle-aged, but it was 20 I wanted,
the youth and the free spirit.
I was retired, but it was middle-age I wanted,
the presence of mind without limitations.
My life was over, and I never got what I wanted.

My point is this: Don't wish your life away. Enjoy every minute God gives you here on this earth. Live every day as if it's your last. Ask God to show you your purpose, to recognize and maximize the talents He has placed within you, and to use them for His glory. When you start living this way, you'll be much happier. If you think you have it bad, I encourage you to visit a chemo room. I spoke at a church recently and after I had finished, a lady came up to me crying and said she was exactly like that. She said she would always say she couldn't wait for Thanksgiving so she would have time off work. Then Thanksgiving came, and her mother died. She said instead of spending time with her mother, she had only focused on herself and how she disliked her job, and now she would never again have that opportunity.

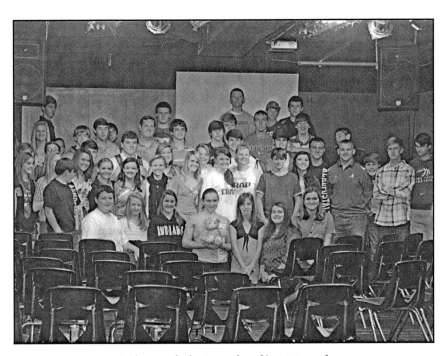

Palmerdale Methodist Youth

Bug Hunting With Ethan

One of the most memorable days I've had was the day my friend Candi Fisher and her sons Trey, eleven, and Ethan, seven, all came over for a visit. Candi, from Piedmont, is married to Jimbo Fisher, head football coach for Florida State University. She has a very busy life being a coach's wife and a mother, but has never forgotten where she came from and visits every Christmas. So what do you get for two boys who live such an exciting life? Their favorite candy of course!

I discovered very quickly that Candi and Jimbo had done a great job raising these boys. They were loving, kind, and very respectful. I also was impressed at how much Trey knew about football. Apparently, the apple **doesn't** fall far from the tree. He wants to be a coach when he grows up; in fact, he already has a play book he's compiled. I don't have any doubt he will someday become a great man and an amazing coach. During their visit in 2010, his mother noticed Ethan was lethargic and not feeling well. When they returned to Florida, the doctor did blood work and discovered he had Fanconi Anemia.

At the present time, Ethan is doing well. I told Ethan when he came to Piedmont that I'd take him on a most excellent bug hunt. When I worked at the daycare, one of the things the children enjoyed more than anything was going on bug hunts. Yes, I know it sounds crazy, but I enjoyed it also. Seeing the children discovering and learning about nature for the first time was so rewarding for me. When Candi told me they were coming for a visit, I looked everywhere for all the cool bug hunting supplies, and the next day Candi dropped Ethan off for our most excellent adventure.

We had garden tools and an old mason jar because these the original bug hunting supplies just can't be beat. We have Cane trees everywhere behind our house. Nathan and Chelsea used to play in them when they were little. Of course, that is where Ethan and I started our bug hunt. The Canes and I have grown much larger than we were when Nathan and Chelsea were younger; I could barley squeeze through them. It was hard to believe that this precious, vibrant little boy has a rare disease that wanted to take his life. Candi told me that one day as she and Ethan were walking into the football stadium, he asked her if he was sick. She asked why he asked her that, and he said his classmates at school told him. He said, "I don't feel sick." This is why I love to be around children. They aren't negative and don't complain. I will always treasure that priceless day. My prayer is that Ethan Alexander Fisher will live a very long and blessed life.

Jeremiah 29:11
New International Version (NIV)

¹¹ For I know the plans I have for you," declares the LORD, "plans to prosper you and not to harm you, plans to give you hope and a future.

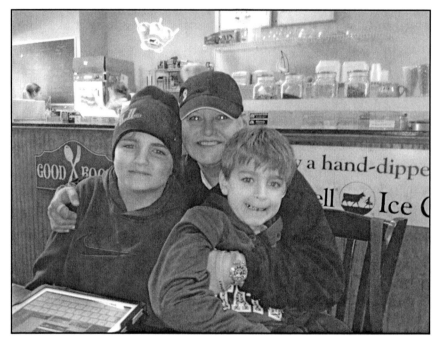

Trey and Ethan

AT THE END OF YOUR ROPE?
THINK YOU JUST CAN'T COPE?
KICK CANCER'S BUTT WITH A
BIG DOSE OF HOPE!

The Holidays

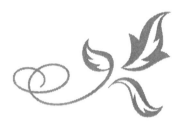

As I've said before. I love Thanksgiving and Christmas. However, that first year without Grandmother, I was very sad; I really wasn't even excited about putting up decorations. I have heard it said that grief is the price we pay for love. As I get older, I realize how much better it will be in Heaven; not only is Jesus there, but I will have treasures there also.

I was surprised one day when I was leaving radiation to have received a call from a man that works for the City of Piedmont. He asked me if I would be one of the grand marshals for the Christmas parade. Needless to say, I was humbled to be considered. My hometown has been so supportive of me and my family. I can't imagine living in a big city where no one knows who you are.

Alyse Radar, a six year old with a rare condition called porphyria, and Kelly Johnson, also a breast cancer survivor, were the other two people to be sharing the spotlight as grand marshals with me. The parade committee was to find us a vehicle to ride on, but when Randa found out about it, nothing but a pink Cadillac would do. By golly, she and Becky found one. Tammy Steed, a lady who sells Mary Kay had a pink Cadillac and said she'd be honored to drive Alyse, Kelly, and me.

My last radiation treatment was December 19. What a great early Christmas present. I had my PET and bone scan done before my last treatment. The bone scan showed a spot on my seventh rib on my left side. The PET scan showed no tumors. My insurance would not approve a CT scan of my chest until Dr. Spremulli called and explained to them that a spot was on my rib, and PET scans are not always accurate finding things in the chest wall.

Waiting for tests and test results is the worst part of having cancer. Finally, I had the CT scan. Kay called and told me it's complicated and the doctor needed to see me the next day. *Really?* I told her I didn't need someone to hold my hand and sit in a comfortable chair, and to please just tell me. She said she couldn't, so, of course I knew it was cancer.

Curtis was with me the following day. The first thing she asked was how I was doing. I said, "I don't know, you tell me!" She said my rib was ok **but –** that is never a good thing to hear in an oncology office- the scan showed two small spots on my right lung. Of course I said, **CRAP!** I asked if it could be damage from radiation. Immediately she said no. Once again I said, **CRAP!** She said the good news was they were very small, three and five millimeters. Of course, I wanted them out! She called the radiologist to see if they were big enough to biopsy, and he said no. **CRAP!** She also said I couldn't have surgery. I would do chemo and have another scan in three months. I said to her, "Look, Dr. Spremulli. I don't have time for this again. I'm writing a book, going and speaking everywhere. I have a

5K mud run in March. I am going to a Tim McGraw concert, and a book tour in the summer!"

She looked at me and smiled. **CRAP!** That would be the first time I'd start treatment without having something taken off or out. I met with Dr. Johnson the next day to schedule having a port put in. I was surprised I still had a place to put one. It was my fourth port.

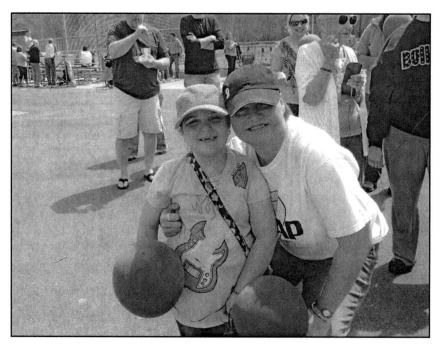

Alyse and me

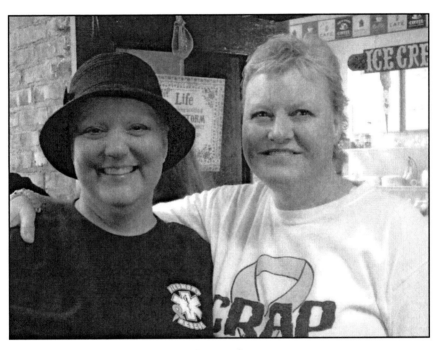

Kelly and me

'LIFO"SUCTION

A MAGNIFICENT
"YOU"
MUST START FROM WITHIN,
TO RECOGNIZE NEGATIVES
IS HOW IT BEGINS,
NEGATIVE PEOPLE,
PLACES AND THINGS,
THE NEGATIVE THOUGHTS
AND THE FEELINGS
THEY BRING,
LIPOSUCTION
REMOVES NASTY FAT,
IT'S KIND OF THE SAME
WITH LIFE'S BAD
THIS &THATS,
ONE BY ONE
JUST REMOVE
ALL THE BAD FROM
YOUR LIFE,
YOU DON'T NEED A DOC
OR A SURGICAL KNIFE,
SO BEGIN YOUR PROCEDURE
WITHOUT INTERRUPTION,
FOCUS ON SMILES,
CALL IT "LIFO"SUCTION!

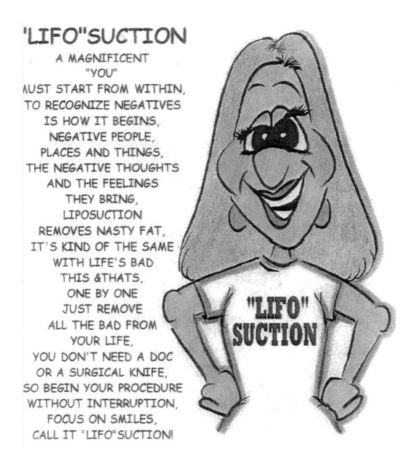

Swollen Lip and Black Eye

My arrival time for having my port inserted was 6:30 a.m., but having done this three other times, I knew that there is no need to stress myself by being on time. Curtis and I arrived at the hospital at 6:30-ish, was directed to my cubical, and started the drill. I put on my gown and waited. Finally, at 9:30 they came to get me. I'm still amazed at anesthesia: One second you are joking with the anesthesiologist, and the next you're waking up in recovery.

I think I fell off the table, or the light above me fell, because my bottom lip was swollen, my left eyelid was black, and I had a terrible headache. Because I had had MRSA and a blood clot on the left side of my neck, Dr Johnson was forced to put the port on the right side, where I had had two already. Consequently, this one would be higher up, and quite uncomfortable. There is nothing like having a tube in your jugular vein! We got home at 2 p.m. I took my pain medicine, got an ice pack for my head and slept the rest of the day. My first chemo treatment was to start in one week.

My Fourth Recurrence, and My Third, and Hopefully Last, Battle with Chemo

It was February 1, 2013. Chemo Day. Proclaiming this and each subsequent Friday for the next four months as "Crap Friday," I asked that everyone wear their crap shirts. When I arrived for my treatment, I was already feeling nervous and nauseated. Having had such a difficult experience with my former chemo tour, I found myself thinking of unpleasant possibilities. My nurse Jackie started to flush my port; it had sludge. *Crap!* She was as gentle as she could be and finally she got it to flush. Even though I had peppermint and gum in my mouth, I could still taste the saline.

I walked into the chemo room and found myself there with only two others. Usually it was full. I made my way to my favorite recliner, the one near the snacks and refrigerator. I told Chris, my chemo nurse, I was in desperate need of a sedative and something for nausea. Thank goodness the treatment would only take thirty minutes. That time I was only to get the chemo drug Gemzar. The chemo nurse started telling me about all the side effects of Gemzar, and once again I was in disbelief that

I was having to go through this, again, and wondering if my body could tolerate more poison. Suddenly my fearful thoughts were interrupted by my phone: my friends were sending me pictures of themselves in their Crap shirts. I felt blanketed by their prayers, and I was powerfully reminded of God's message to me, instructing me to write and speak. Asking God for strength, I began writing in my journal.

By the time my treatment was finished, the room had started to fill with other victims of this horrible disease, and I prayed for them and thanked God that I was able to leave without the help of a wheel chair or someone having to hold me up. My story, thus far, has been one of both pain and pleasure; consequently, I am reminded of this question from Job 2:10: "Shall we indeed accept good from God and not accept adversity?" No, God planned our lives to provide us choices to make; our responses make us either a casualty or a champion. Therefore, my sincere hope for you is that if you are given "CRAP" in life, you will use it to make you better, not bitter.

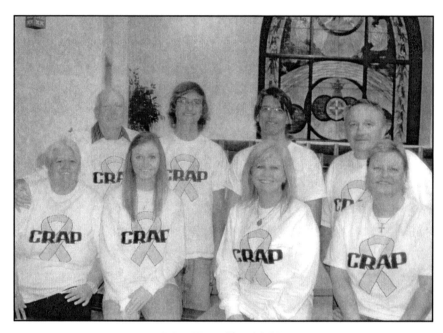

My Family 2013

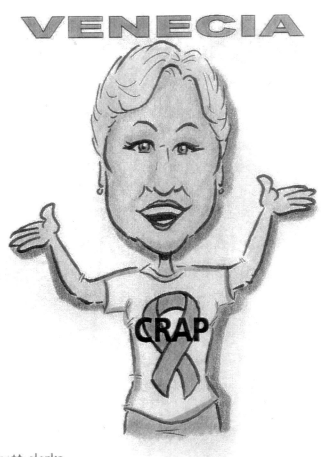

scott clarke

Author Contact Information

If you are interested in having Venecia come speak at your church or event, or you want to purchase a CRAP shirt; you can contact her at veneciabutler@gmail.com

To see where the crap shirts have been, visit Venecia's Facebook page – Venecia Benefield Butler

V Foundation

I am excited to announce the formation of the **"V Foundation",** an incorporated, non-profit organization, whose purpose is to provide aid, support, and comfort to cancer patients and their families. I personally have experienced the seemingly endless misery of cancer treatment; consequently, my goal is to brighten the day of those in treatment by sharing my faith and love, and seeing that chemo rooms have portable DVD players, and lots of comedy's for the patients to watch, and care packages with gas cards and things that helped me get through chemo. Please contact me if you are interested in investing time or money in this very worthy and much needed cause.

Contact Information:
veneciabutler@gmail.com
V Foundation
P.O. Box 572
Piedmont, Alabama
36272

Scott Clark
Artist/writer/activist/father
WWW.CRABBYCARDS.COM'

Scott Clarke, artist, writer, production, packaging and marketing guy of Crabby Cards. This is a small business I run from my bedroom at home, my daughter took my little home office for a playroom! I began this work just a few years ago with the intent combining my artistic abilities and my own brand of humor, which tends to be a bit "Crabby" I have since designed greeting cards on subjects such as aging, golf, navy football(an Annapolis thing!), corvettes and much more. Though I enjoy the challenge of combining subject matter with artwork, I have also craved the opportunity to help others in some way with my work.

Which brings about the question quite frequently asked of me, "Why Breast Cancer Awareness?" About the same time I began Crabby Cards my Mother-In-law was battling a second time with breast cancer. I looked on and felt helpless, I wanted so badly to help in some way, which I believe is a feeling men everywhere go through when confronted with this disease, even though 1% of yearly diagnosed cases are men. Then my ex-wife and her sister were tested and found to carry the mutated gene which increases their chances of developing breast cancer. My ex-wife and her sister have both opted for precautionary surgeries, and then my concern deepened for the fate of my ten year old daughter whose breasts had just begun to develop my fatherly fear and need to protect her set in; I wondered how could I possibly make a difference?

It was about this time that a friend of mine Kim, who is involved with the local "Save the Boobies" foundation, approached me and asked me if I would design some greeting cards to help promote a breast cancer awareness event they had coming up. I was immediately on board and felt this was my calling! It has since been an amazing, educational and bittersweet journey. I have met women with courage I could only dream of having, survivors with stories that are moving beyond what I could ever put in a greeting card. Women that continue to fill me with inspiration that flows through me and on to paper.

I try very hard to incorporate every aspect I can in to my work, from the importance of 'Early Detection" to the "Spiritual and Supportive" needs we all have as human beings. Giving women a chance to share compassion AND very important information. Some of the styles rhyme and some don't, some celebrities have been incorporated in to the some styles, subjects from beauty pageants to American Idol have been incorporated in, and the styles range from young, old, birthdays, get well, thank you and more, but all aim toward an attempt to share in support and awareness. In addition, my work is always open to change, suggestions, tweaking, etc.! I also do my best to make my work affordable so that organizations are able to raise funds for their specific goals to be met.

What is Fanconi Anemia?

Fanconi anemia (FA) is an orphan disease and rare medical condition affecting about one in 131,000 people, occurs equally in males and females and all ethnic groups.

Patients with FA can have a variety of health issues including shortness, dark and light areas of skin, abnormalities of the arms and hands, kidney problems, heart defects, hearing problems and others.

Some patients have no physical findings, but nearly all will have a decline in their blood counts over time, eventually leading to bone marrow failure.

While the average life expectancy is twenty-five years, an increasing number of patients are living into their 30s and beyond. There is no cure for the disease itself, but treatments are available for the bone marrow failure associated with FA.

Until recently, the most common reason for shortened survival was due to marrow failure. When the marrow fails, it no longer makes the needed numbers of red blood cells (anemia), white blood cells (increasing the risk of infection) and platelets (increasing the risk of bleeding).

Today, a bone marrow transplant is the only treatment of bone marrow failure. While bone marrow transplant is risky, discoveries at the University of Minnesota have markedly improved survival for this specific disease. In 1995, only one out of every seven patients with FA survived an unrelated donor transplant; today, six out of every seven are expected to survive.

FA is something that a person is born with–even if they seem healthy as a baby. The FA genes are responsible for preventing cancer and bone marrow failure by repairing DNA damage that occurs in everyday life (from sun exposure, x-rays, chemicals in our food and surroundings). Without this restorative ability, people with FA have a significantly higher chance of developing certain types of cancers at a much earlier age than the general population.

Understanding how the FA genes work is vitally important to understanding cancer and bone marrow function that impacts everyone in the general population. Research in FA will have far-reaching impact well beyond patients with this rare disease. There is already a long list of connections between FA genes and the DNA repair pathway, including genes that lead to breast, ovarian and cervical cancer susceptibility as well as head and neck cancer, leukemia, lymphoma, and multiple myeloma.

Research in FA has led to the creation of cord blood transplantation and promoted the founding of the National Marrow Donor Program. FA has also taught us about the genes responsible for growth and development, fertility, diabetes and marrow function.

How did Kidz 1st Fund begin?

Kidz 1st Fund was established by Jimbo and Candi Fisher after their younger son, Ethan, was diagnosed with FA in the spring of 2011.

The Fishers launched their public battle against Fanconi anemia on August 5, 2011 in the hopes of improving treatment options, raising national awareness of the disease, and helping to fund research that will lead to a cure.

Ethan's doctors at the University of Minnesota estimate he will need a bone marrow transplant in the next three to five years. Since the Fisher's elder son Trey is not a match, Ethan's transplanted bone marrow will come from an unrelated donor.

Jimbo and Candi Fisher and Kidz 1st Fund support the efforts of the C.W. "Bill" Young Cell Transplantation Program, a federal program that supports bone marrow and cord blood donation and transplantation, by encouraging participation in the national bone marrow registry for Ethan and all patients needing a transplant.

Why the University of Minnesota?

Kidz 1st Fund raises money for Fanconi anemia research at the Fanconi Anemia Comprehensive Care Program at the University of Minnesota's Amplatz Children's Hospital, the single largest treatment center for patients with FA in the country.

The specialists at the University of Minnesota are working relentlessly to find a cure for Fanconi anemia. Most affected with FA will need a transplant of stem cells, derived either from bone marrow or umbilical cord blood, to extend their lives. University of Minnesota physician-scientists performed the world's first successful bone marrow transplant in 1968 and have been blazing new trails in the field since.

Through research, improvements are made each year in treating patients with FA that have changed the survival rate after unrelated donor bone marrow transplant for this disease from less than thirty percent to greater than eighty percent in the last fifteen years.

What are the goals of Kidz 1ˢᵗ Fund?

The Fishers created a fund at the Minnesota Medical Foundation titled "Kidz 1ˢᵗ Fund for Fanconi Anemia Research" in which all proceeds from Kidz 1ˢᵗ Fund are donated.

The purpose of the Fund is to support FA research focused on the development of safer treatments for FA patients with marrow failure, myelodysplastic syndrome, and cancer as well as the identification of new therapeutic approaches for preventing and treating cancers particular to FA.

Donations to Kidz 1ˢᵗ Fund support FA research as directed by Drs. Margaret MacMillan and John Wagner, world renowned FA physicians.

Kidz 1ˢᵗ Fund has an annual financial goal of $500,000 to the University of Minnesota. The initial donation of $500,000 was delivered to the University of Minnesota after just six months of Kidz 1ˢᵗ Fund being in existence. Currently, Kidz 1ˢᵗ Fund has given more than $1,000,000 for FA research.

Contact Information:
Website: www.Kidz1stFund.com
Address: Kidz1stFund
1400 Village Square Boulevard
Suite 3-229

Tallahassee, Florida 32312

Email: info@kidz1stfund.com

Facebook: Kidz1stFund

Twitter: @Kidz1stFund

Tax ID #: 45-4355903

501(c)(3) nonprofit organization

FL REG #: CH36019

Candi Fisher

Chairwoman

Candi@Kidz1stFund.com

Cameron Ulrich

Director of Operations

Cameron@Kidz1stFund.com

850.443.7777

For more information about Fanconi anemia, please visit: www.Fanconi.org

For more information about bone marrow donation, please visit: www.Marrow.org

What is Porphyria?

Alyse Rader is a 6 year old little girl with a rare condition called Porphyria. Alyse has been battling Porphyria for her entire life.

Porphyria is a disease in which her body produces an enzyme called a prophyrin that attacks her red blood cells. It causes them to break down prematurely and the porphyrins land in her joints and cause swelling and pain and can damage her organs causing severe pain. She was finally diagnosed at the age of two thanks to her wonderful pediatrician Chase Thomas who finally believed mom and dad that something wasn't right and that everything had to do with the same thing. After going to Children's Hospital and having twenty-four hour testing and then a liver biopsy, she finally had a name for all the things that were going on.

She starting seeing a specialist in Birmingham and for the first two or three years it seemed that since they had a diagnosis and knew what to stay away from she was doing better. Then, all of the sudden she continued to have problem after problem. If Alyse goes out in the sun she breaks out in a rash and begins to swell and have belly pain. There are certain things she can't eat because it causes her to go into a breakout. Since her diagnosis they have to come to know that her gallbladder is dead, her liver is diseased, her adrenal gland is diseased, she has high blood pressure, severe acid reflux and belly pain from the irritation in her GI tract, she has blank stare seizers, she writes things upside down and backwards when she is in a severe outbreak, she loses short term memory, she has become scared to be around strangers or crowded places. The list continues to grow.

Alyse has been hospitalized too many times to count in the past four years but just in the past year she's spent more time at Children's Hospital than she has at home. For months we were at the hospital at least one week out of every month. On top of being hospitalized so much, she has to wear a backpack with an IV twenty-four hours a day. She has had a PIC line inserted in her arm for IV therapy which got infected so a Broviac central line had to be placed. She's had two lines put in because the first got pulled. The Broviac goes in through her side and is threaded in a vein directly into her heart because she has fluids running so long and so fast that her veins can't handle the rate of fluid.

She is currently battling a GI bleed which will require surgery just to find. She had to have a blood transfusion because of this issue. Children's Hospital has done all they know to do for her so the family is now trying to get her to a Porphyria clinic in Texas. As soon as they can get her records transferred and her insurance on board they will be headed to Texas to see if there is anything that has yet to be tried. Her parents absolutely believe in healing and that God can and will heal her one day!

Porphyria is not a single disease but a group of at least eight disorders that differ considerably from each other. A common feature in all porphyrias is the accumulation in the body of porphyrins or porphyrin precursors. Although these are normal body chemicals, they normally do not accumulate. Precisely which of these chemicals builds up depends on the type of porphyria.

The porphyrias are rare diseases. Taken together, all forms of porphyria afflict fewer than 200,000 people in the United States. Based on European studies, the prevalence of the most common porphyria, porphyria cutanea tarda (PCT), is one in 10,000, the most common acute porphyria, acute intermittent porphyria (AIP), is about one in 20,000, and the most common erythropoietic porphyria, erythropoietic protoporphyria (EPP), is estimated at one in 50,000 to 75,000. Congenital erythropoietic porphyria (CEP) is extremely rare with prevalence estimates of one in 1,000,000 or less. Only six cases of ALAD-deficiency porphyria (ADP) are documented.

Acute Intermittent Porphyria (AIP)

AIP manifests especially in women (due to hormonal influences). Symptoms usually occur as attacks that develop over several hours or days. Abdominal pain, which can be severe, is the most common symptom. Other symptoms may include:

- nausea
- vomiting
- constipation
- pain in the back, arms and legs
- muscle weakness (due to effects on nerves supplying the muscles)
- urinary retention
- palpitation (due to a rapid heart rate and often accompanied by increased blood pressure)
- confusion, hallucinations and seizures
- Blisters develop on sun-exposed areas of the skin, such as the hands and face. The skin in these areas may blister or peel after minor trauma.

Sometimes the level of salt (sodium and chloride) in the blood decreases markedly and contributes to some of these symptoms. Hospitalization is often necessary for acute attacks. Medications for pain, nausea and vomiting, and close observation are generally required.

A high intake of glucose or other carbohydrates can help suppress disease activity and can be given by vein or by mouth.

Hepatoerythropoietic Porphyria (HEP)

This very rare type of Porphyria is also due to a deficiency of uroporphyrinogen decarboxylase (UROD). The enzyme deficiency is inherited as an autosomal recessive trait. The manifestations of HEP resemble CEP, with symptoms of skin blistering usually beginning in infancy. Porphyrins are increased in bone marrow and red blood cells, in contrast to PCT, as well as liver, plasma, urine and feces

CPSIA information can be obtained at www.ICGtesting.com
Printed in the USA
LVOW120449080713

341639LV00004B/8/P